Stephanie
CLAIRMONT, RD

The
IBS
MASTER
PLAN

First Published 2013 by Stephanie Clairmont, RD

www.StephanieClairmont.com

Copyright @ 2013 Stephanie Clairmont

All rights reserved

No part of this publication may be reproduced or distributed in any form or by any means, electronic or mechanical, or stored in a database or retrieval system, without prior written permission from the publisher.

ISBN: 978-1500762506

This book is a general guide only and is not intended to replace skill, knowledge, and experience of a qualified medical professional. It is recommended by the author that all those experiencing digestive distress seek the advice of their doctor first. The information in this book is not intended to treat, diagnose, cure, or prevent any disease, including digestive problems.

The tools presented in this book have been created using scientific literature on the various nutrition concepts such as the low FODMAP diet, fibre, exercise, etc. Each person is individual and may have different food allergies and/or intolerances. This book has been designed to use along with guidance from your doctor and/or registered dietitian. We recommend you work with a medical professional to help you figure out the best diet for you and your digestive health concerns.

We cannot be responsible for any hazards, loss, or damage that may occur as a result of use of this book.

Design: Stasia Blanco
Editor: Julie Pickar
Writers: Stephanie Clairmont, MHSc, RD and Bina Moore, MSW

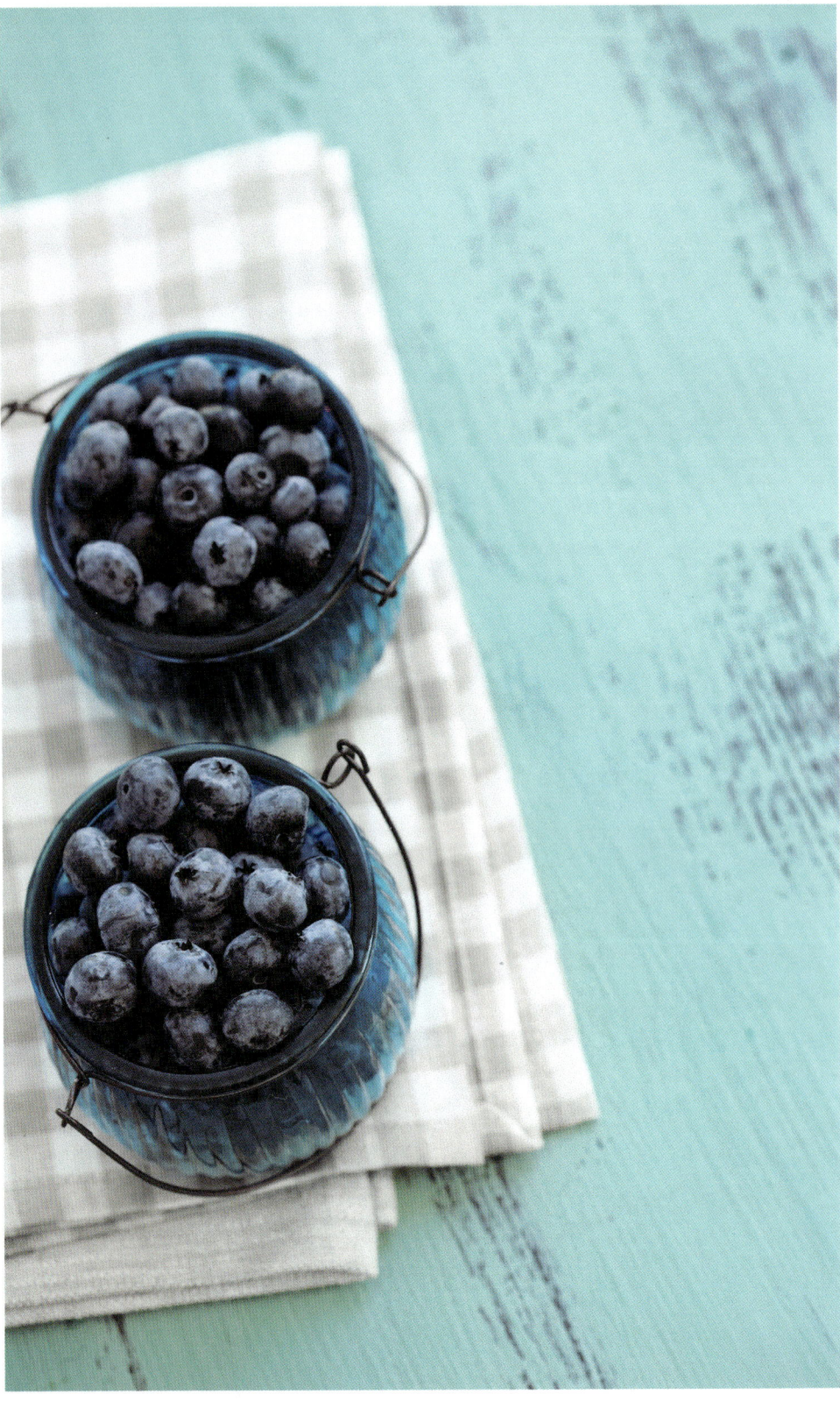

Contents

Chapter One — 8

- Introduction — 11
- The Master Plan — 15
- Step 1: Eat for Good Digestion — 17
- Step 2: Eat Foods that are Low in FODMAPs — 20
- Step 3: Get Your Fibre! — 35
- Step 4: Make Every Day a Healthy Eating Day — 42
- Step 5: Make a Plan for Success — 44
- Step 6: Keep a Food & Symptom Journal — 49
- Step 7: Be Active Every Day — 55
- Step 8: Work on Mind-Body Balance — 57
- Recommended Resources — 69

Chapter Two — 70

Breakfast — 72

- Amazing Oatmeal — 75
- Sensational Smoothies — 76
- Tasty Toast Balanced Breakfast — 78
- Fabulous French Toast and Pancakes — 80

Soups, Salads, and Sides — 86

- Stupendous Superfood Minestrone — 88
- Hearty Wholesome Harvest Soup — 90
- Roasted Red Pepper Pasta Salad — 92
- Lemon Dill Tuna Pasta Salad — 94
- Roasted Vegetable Lentil Salad — 96
- Leafy Italian Salad with Quinoa — 98

Simple Rice Paper Salad Rolls 100
Spanish Quinoa Side Salad 102
Protein Power Side Salad 103
Lemon Arugula Side Salad 104
Caprese Side Salad 105
Spring Pea Risotto 106
Grilled Vegetables and Potatoes 108

Meatless Meals 110

Vegetarian Vegetable Bolognese 112
Smokey Tempeh and Lentil Chili 114
Spinach Salad Bowls with Tempeh Bacon 116
Tempeh Taco Salad 118
Crunchy Cornmeal-Crusted Tofu in Collard Wraps with Quinoa 120
Easy Lentil Quesadillas 122
Pan-Fried Cod with Vegetable Quinoa 124
Breaded Cod with Rice Pilaf 126
Grilled Pickerel 128
Salmon en Papillotte 130
Salmon Kale Salad Sandwiches 132
Corn-Crusted Trout 134
Roasted Red Pepper Tuna Quinoa Cakes 136
Shrimp Burgers with Tomato Avocado Salsa 138
Perfect Peanut Noodle Bowl 140

Meat and Poultry 142

Sesame Chicken Lettuce Tacos with Rice Noodles 144
Curry Chicken Salad Lettuce Wraps 146
Pineapple Chicken Salad Bowl with Rice Noodles 148
Roasted Chicken Breast 150
Grilled Flank Steak 152
Chicken Cotoletta with Roasted Carrots and Green Beans 154
Pan-Fried Chicken Pasta with Fresh Tomato Sauce 156
Classic Chicken Corn Fajitas 158
Beef and Vegetable Burritos 160

Chili Chicken Stuffed Peppers 162
Simple Beef Burgers 164
The Best Turkey Burgers 166

Chapter Three 168

Meal Plan Week One 170
Grocery List Week One 172
Meal Plan Week Two 174
Grocery List Week Two 176
Meal Plan Week Three 178
Grocery List Week Three 180
Meal Plan Week Four 182
Grocery List Week Four 184
Pantry List 186

Make Your Own Meal Plan Tool 188

Make-Your-Own Meal Plan 191
6 Meal Planning Strategies 193
Snack Options 195
Make-Your-Own Meal Plan Template 196
My Meal Plan 198
About the Author 200

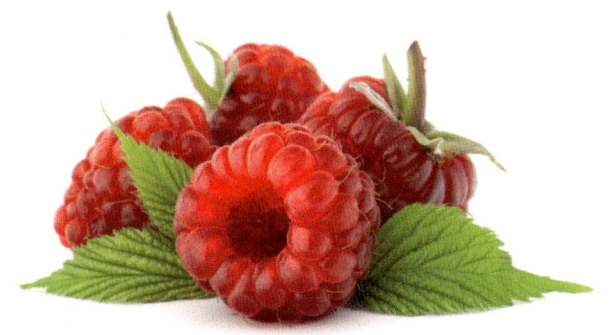

Chapter One

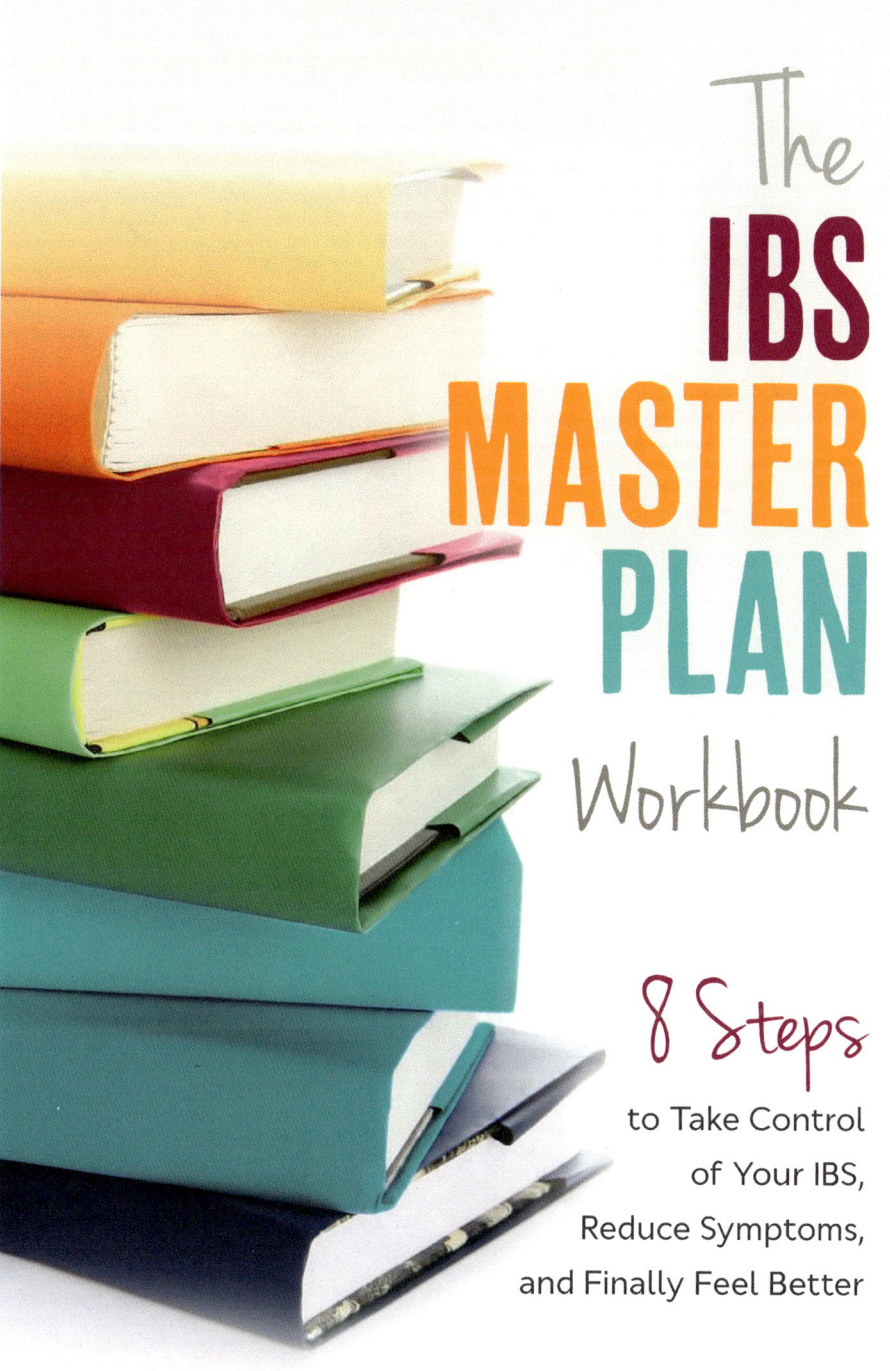

The IBS MASTER PLAN Workbook

8 Steps to Take Control of Your IBS, Reduce Symptoms, and Finally Feel Better

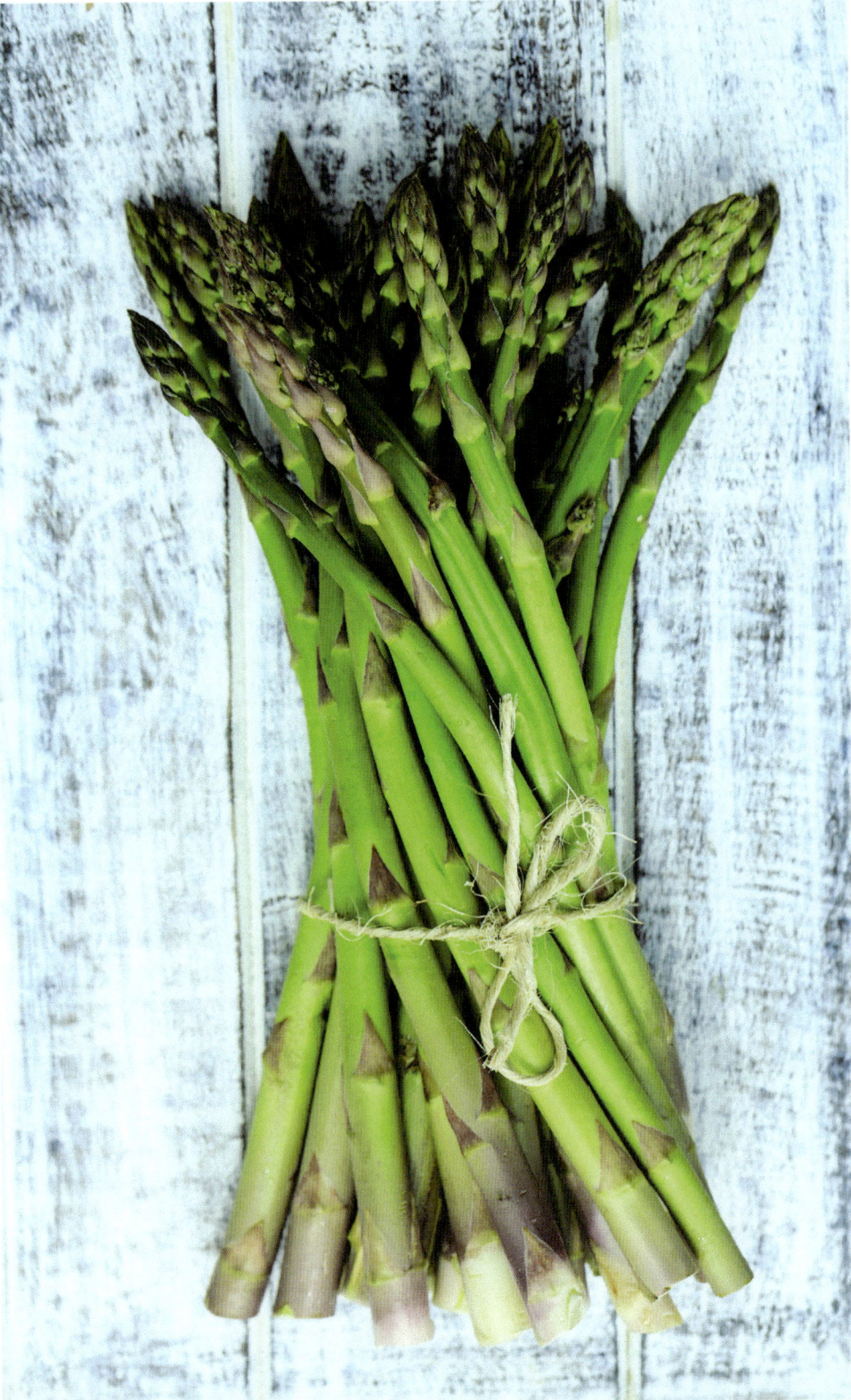

Introduction

Irritable Bowel Syndrome (IBS) is a functional gastrointestinal disorder (FGID) that is common in people around the world. The Canadian Digestive Health Foundation estimates five million people currently suffer from IBS in Canada alone. IBS is classified with abdominal pain or discomfort along with several other symptoms that may or may not include gas, bloating, distention of the abdomen, diarrhea, and/or constipation. It can involve problems with how food moves through the digestive system as well as increase individual sensitivity to foods. The exact cause of IBS is unknown at this time, but it is believed to be related both psychologically and physiologically to the body and may involve more than one factor.

There are several recommended diets that have been used to treat IBS over the past decade. Although they differ in types of foods allowed and restricted, they do share some similarities. One diet, the low FODMAP diet, has shown results through research that it can help to treat IBS. This diet was developed in 1999 by a leading dietitian in digestive health, Dr. Sue Shepherd in Australia. Through her PhD research and along with the team at Monash University, they have developed this diet as an effective, evidence-based treatment for people suffering from symptoms of IBS. The research that this diet is beneficial for other types of digestive conditions is slim to-date, but there are many anecdotal stories of clients that have been reducing FODMAP foods and have experienced digestive symptom relief.

In my own practice, at the Clairmont Digestive Clinic, I have seen clients with diagnosed IBS, Inflammatory Bowel Disease (IBD), and undiagnosed digestive symptoms (like excessive gas and bloating) decrease digestive symptoms by changing their diet to one that is much easier on the digestive system. That said, each person is unique and will benefit from various treatments regarding their health. Food can affect everyone differently as well, so foods that bother one individual with IBS may not cause symptoms in another. At the Clairmont Digestive Clinic we practice a mind-body approach and incorporate strategies for coping with stress and anxiety into the treatment of IBS. We believe that diet and good nutrition are key to the health of an individual. However, through a holistic mind-body approach, we can help people feel much better and reduce long-term suffering from symptoms of digestive distress helping them to take control of their lives.

How to Use This Book

The IBS Master Plan contains a workbook section, which is meant to provide those suffering with IBS and other digestive issues the information needed to help improve symptoms. There are eight main strategies that when combined work well to improve digestive health. By avoiding foods that are not digested well and adding other strategies to make healthy lifestyle changes, you can see improvement in your digestive health. At the Clairmont Digestive Clinic, we have found an improvement in over 80% of our clients that follow this plan. The IBS Master Plan also includes a cookbook section with recipes that are low in FODMAPs. You can use these recipes to eat delicious food while avoiding foods that will cause digestive distress. There are also meal plans to show you how to plan for a balanced and healthy week.

It is recommended to implement as many of the dietary and lifestyle guidelines in the eight steps for at least one month. Make sure you track your progress to see how your symptoms are changing. After one month, depending on how you're feeling, you may start to re-introduce various foods. This is where it is best to work with a registered dietitian to help you identify patterns and understand what to do next.

The IBS Master Plan works best along with professional expertise of health care professionals for optimal healing. It is highly recommended that if you have been diagnosed with IBS, IBD, Celiac Disease, or another condition, that you work with a registered dietitian and social worker, psychologist, or therapist that specializes in digestive health. The IBS Master Plan provides you with all the information and tools to help you identify triggers and start to work on reducing them, but because every case of IBS is different, you will see the most success with an individual approach.

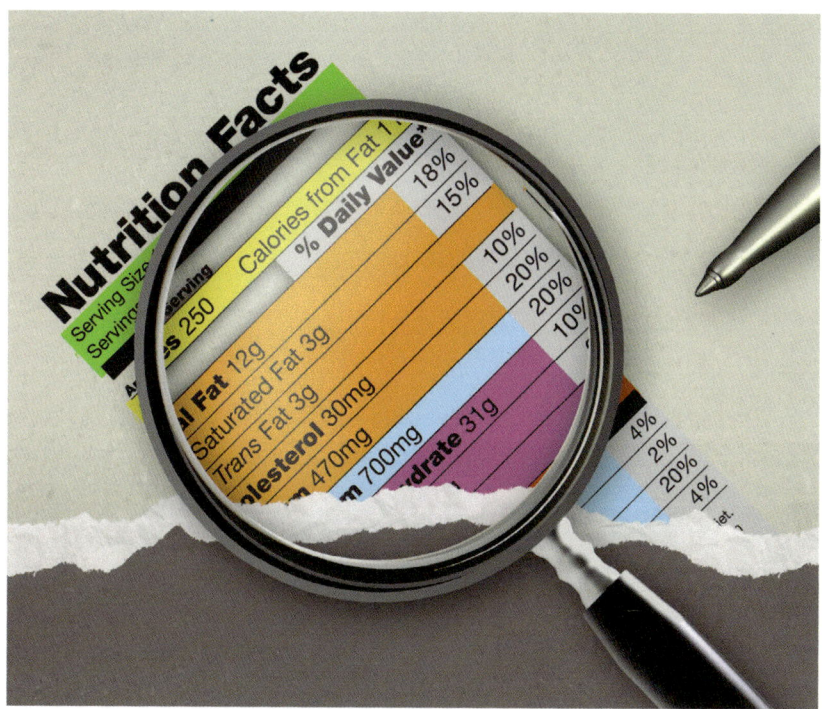

A registered dietitian can help create a custom approach for you. Digestive nutrition and health is complicated and each individual requires a modified approach. What works for one person, may not work for another. The world of food and nutrition is changing constantly, so working with a registered dietitian can help you navigate your way through nutrition advice, food labels, recipes, and meal plans to help you feel better faster.

One of the underlying potential causes of IBS is stress and anxiety, and particularly the way we cope with them in daily life. It's important in the journey of digestive symptom relief to consider this and adopt a mindfulness approach when looking at your symptoms. Consider working with a mental health professional like a social worker, psychologist, or therapist to discover underlying sources of stress, other triggers like places or people, and to learn ways to cope with day-to-day issues.

Much love, health, & good eating,
Stephanie Clairmont, MHSc, RD

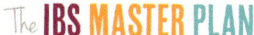
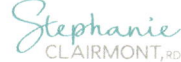

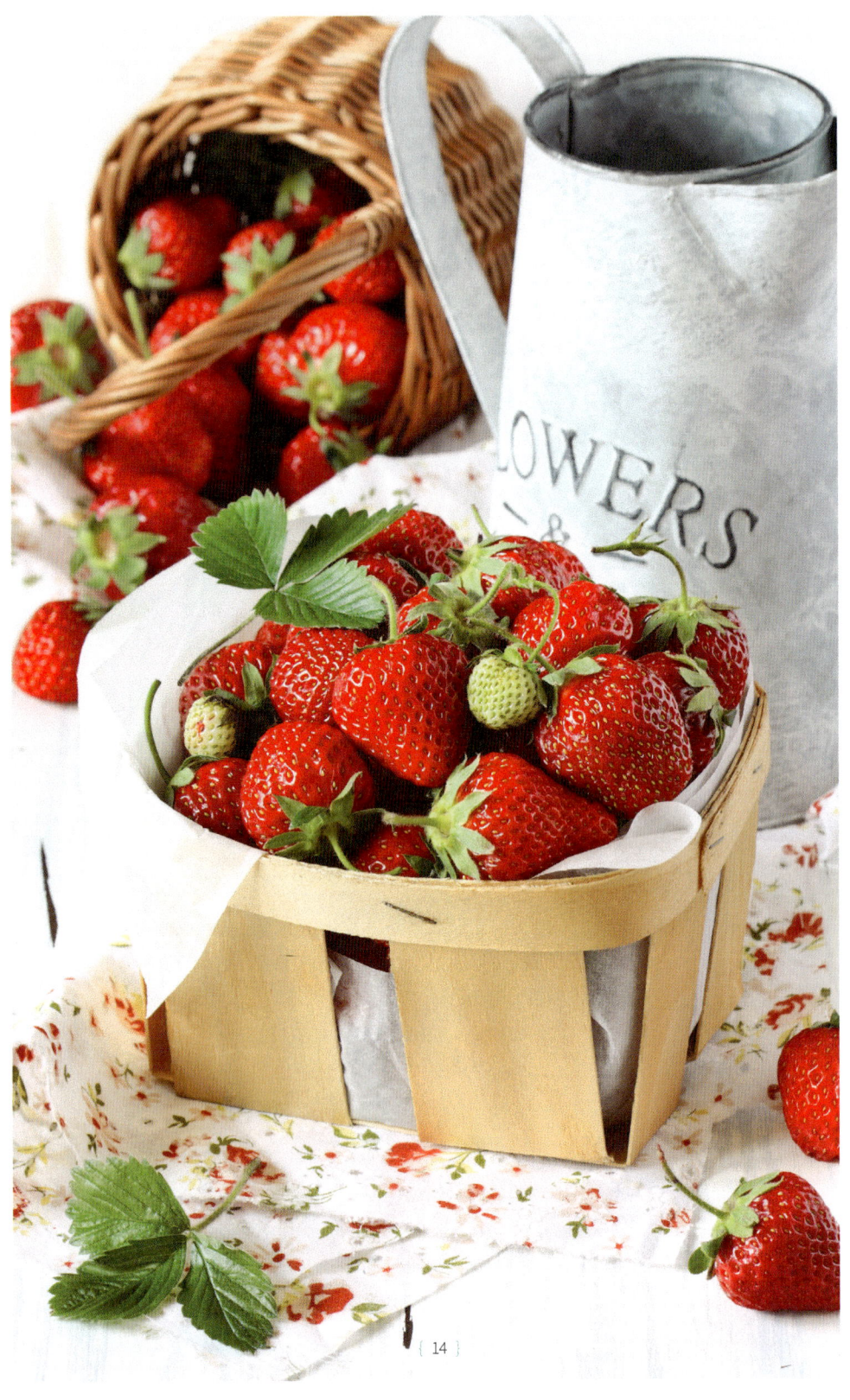

The Master Plan

Here are the 8 strategies to help you take control of your IBS, reduce symptoms, and finally feel better. This is truly a lifestyle prescription for digestive healing and has been developed through research, evidence-based protocols, and clinical expertise in practice. It is recommended to follow this plan for 4 to 8 weeks fairly strictly to see the best results. Then you can start to re-introduce foods one at a time to see what may be causing you symptoms.

1. **EAT FOR GOOD DIGESTION.** Avoid trigger foods, include foods that are easy to digest, drink enough fluid, and eat throughout the day.

2. **EAT FOODS THAT ARE LOW IN FODMAPS.**

3. **INCLUDE ENOUGH FIBRE.** Ensure you spread fibre throughout the day at meals and snacks, and do not consume large quantities at one time.

4. **EAT HEALTHY.** Include many foods that are good for you and balance out meals and snacks throughout the day with real, wholesome, seasonal food.

5. **PLAN AHEAD.** Choose recipes to include in a weekly meal plan and stick to it.

6. **TRACK.** Keep a Food & Symptom Journal to record your progress for 2 to 4 months, while making diet and lifestyle changes.

7. **ADD IN EXERCISE.** Daily exercise helps your digestive system work properly.

8. **BALANCE OUT THE MIND AND BODY.** Reflect on stress and anxiety triggers in your life and implement strategies to improve coping.

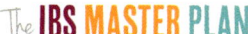 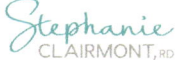

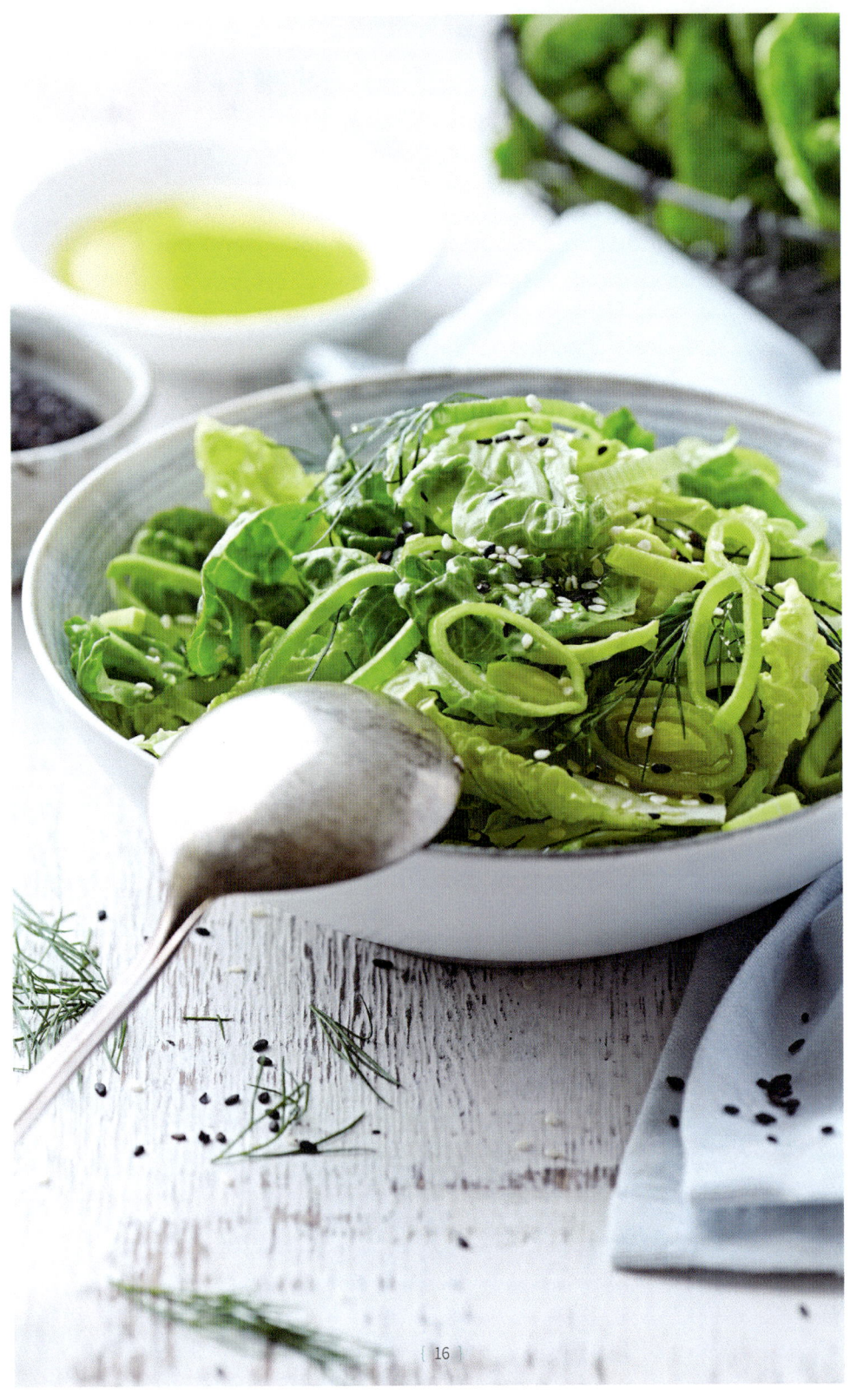

Step 1:
Eat for Good Digestion

When you're experiencing digestive distress, it's best to do everything possible to give your gut a break. Here we take into account all recommendations for digestive health and the reduction of IBS symptoms like gas, bloating, abdominal discomfort, diarrhea, and constipation. Follow these guidelines for overall healthy digestion.

1. Include more **cooked vegetables** than raw in your diet. Raw vegetables take extra work for your gut to breakdown and can cause symptoms of IBS. Reduce or eliminate raw vegetables for 4 to 8 weeks while implementing this plan. Enjoy cooked vegetables in soups, stews, stir-fry, casseroles, pasta dishes, salads, and as side dishes. To include raw vegetables, puree vegetables into smoothies or juices as a great way to get all the nutrients you need without consuming large amounts of raw vegetable fibre.

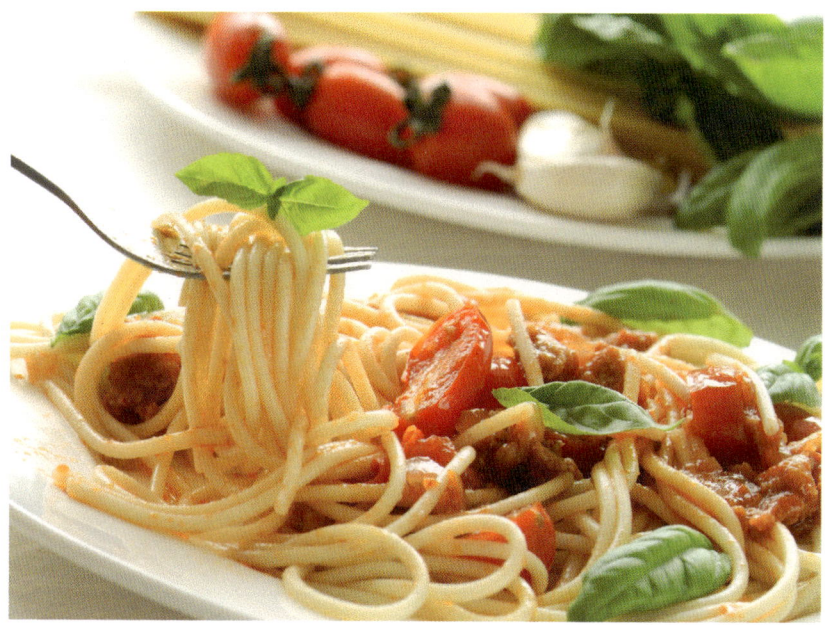

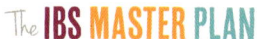

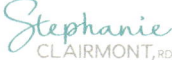

2. Some ingredients stimulate the digestive tract, encouraging the gut to move. These foods can be beneficial for those with constipation, but if you are suffering from diarrhea, loose stool, or multiple bowel movements (more than 3) each day, it may be beneficial to **avoid gut stimulants.** By avoiding these, you will give the bowel more time to digest, which can reduce the above mentioned symptoms. Gut stimulants include foods that contain caffeine, nicotine, and alcohol.

3. Several foods can increase gas production in the gut. Not only is excessive gas uncomfortable and embarrassing, but this can also cause stomach discomfort, bloating, excessive rumbling sounds, and flatulence. To reduce these symptoms, **avoid foods that stimulate gas production,** which includes:

   - Lactose
   - Sugar alcohols—mannitol, xylitol, and sorbitol
   - Carbonated beverages
   - Beans and lentils
   - Sulphurous vegetables—onions, garlic, cabbage, Brussels sprouts, asparagus, cauliflower, and broccoli

4. How you eat and the timing of your meals through the day is absolutely critical to healthy digestion and can directly affect digestive distress symptoms. Consume meals and snacks at regular times through the day in a relaxed atmosphere. **Have a meal or snack every 3 to 4 hours.** Always sit and enjoy your meals without distraction to allow your body to be calm and focus on digestion.

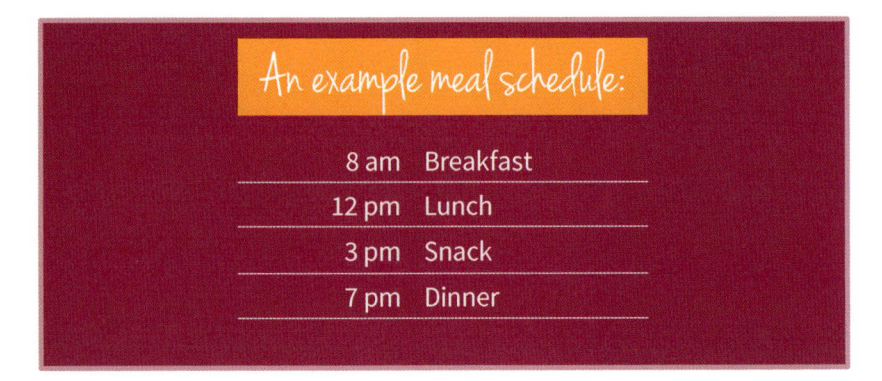

An example meal schedule:

8 am	Breakfast
12 pm	Lunch
3 pm	Snack
7 pm	Dinner

Avoid consuming food less than two hours apart to allow your digestive track a break. Scheduling two hours without snacking or drinking calories (like coffee with milk and sugar) allows the migrating motor complex, or cleansing wave to work well and move food through the gut before the next meal or snack arrives.

5. Drink your fluid. Include at least **2 to 3 L of water every day.** Water helps to keep things moving along and balance out the acidity of the gut. However, it's important that you avoid drinking large amounts of fluids with meals. It may actually be best for your body to not drink at all with meals and to schedule your fluid intake between eating. Excess fluid during meals for some individuals can affect the acidity of the gut and the overall digestive process.

6. **Herbal tea** can be beneficial for digestion, especially after a big meal or one that you've included foods on that are known symptom triggers for your body. There are several herbal teas available on the market that may aid in digestion. Consider purchasing a loose leaf tea from a tea speciality store so you know it's fresh. You can also make your own with fresh herbs. Although many herbal ingredients have all kinds of beneficial properties, the three best ingredients to help aid in digestion and soothe digestive discomfort are **ginger, fennel, and peppermint.**

> **Tip:**
>
> If you're away from home, travelling, or eating in a restaurant—ask for one bag peppermint tea and one bag chamomile in a large mug of hot water. This combination is a great stomach soother when you're out in the world.

7. Doing things to increase the amount of air in the stomach can increase discomfort and gas production. To prevent this, avoid drinking carbonated beverages, drinking with a straw, and chewing gum.

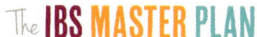
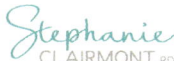

Step 2: Eat Foods that are Low in FODMAPs

What is FODMAPs?

FODMAPs is an abbreviation that stands for:
Fermentable **O**ligosaccharides, **D**isaccharides, **M**onosaccharides, and **P**olyols.

These are complex names for a group of carbohydrates that can be poorly absorbed by the body. Many individuals cannot digest these molecules and for those with IBS, symptoms are experienced to a much greater extent. When FODMAPs are poorly absorbed they can create gas in the gut which then contributes to other symptoms such as bloating, abdominal distension, pain or discomfort, diarrhea, and/or constipation.

These types of foods have been discussed in IBS treatment diets for decades, however the term FODMAP and the Low FODMAP diet has been designed by the team at Monash University. An exclusion diet like this is most effective when followed under the supervision of a registered dietitian so that you can be sure you are getting all the nutrients needed while avoiding trigger foods. The exclusion diet should be followed for 4 to 12 weeks depending on the individual and symptom relief experienced. After this time, if symptom relief has been experienced, it is time to enter into the **reintroduction phase.** If you experience NO SYMPTOM IMPROVEMENT—you do not need to continue to follow this diet. Seek advice from your doctor immediately.

During the reintroduction phase, one food should be reintroduced at a time in a quantity that would be normal for you, for example a half an apple or one whole apple might be a normal serving. Then wait 48 hours to see if any symptoms occur. Keep track of what's happening to your body in this phase with your food and symptom journal. If no symptoms occur than try this challenge food again and then wait another 48 hours. If no symptoms are experienced after two introductions of this food, you can consider this food as safe and add it back to your diet. You will get the best results during this reintroduction phase when working with a digestive dietitian as food is complex and an expert can help you understand ingredients and patterns. It is highly recommended to work with your doctor first to gain a diagnosis of IBS and follow the exclusion diet along with a registered dietitian.

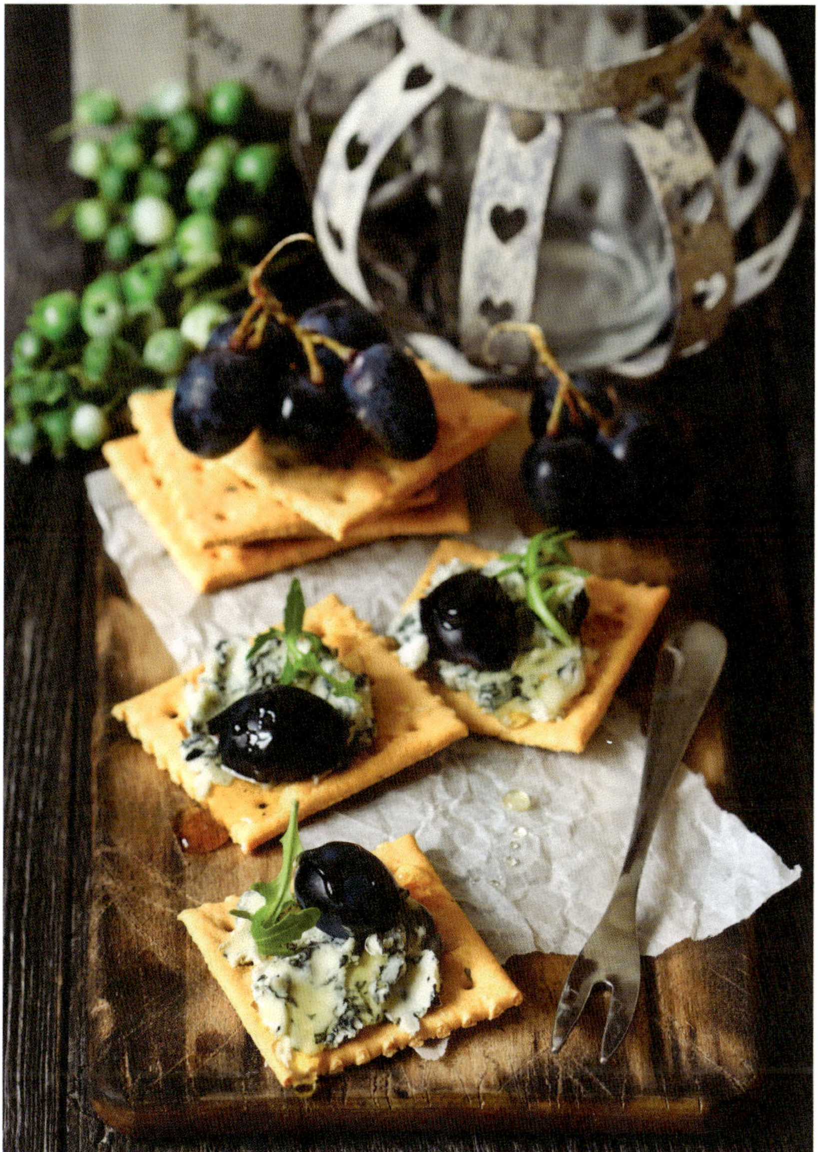

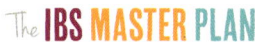 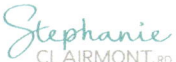

FODMAP Food List

Adapted from the Monash University Low FODMAP App for Iphone.

VEGETABLES

Enjoy several servings of vegetables every day as snacks or with a meal. Vegetables are packed with vitamins and minerals and are low in calories so they are key to keeping you healthy. Include leafy green vegetables daily in smoothies, sauces, stir-fry, and in salad. Raw vegetables, even those that are low in FODMAPs, may be difficult for some people to digest. Be mindful of this and listen to your body. You may want to consume raw vegetables in small servings and focus on including more cooked vegetables in your eating plan.

Low in FODMAPs

Include a variety of these foods every day

Arugula	Eggplant	Red pepper
Alfalfa	Endive leaves	Potatoes
Bean sprouts	Fennel bulb	Pumpkin
Green beans	Fennel leaves	Radish
Bok choy	Ginger root	Spinach, baby
Brussel sprouts	Kale	Spring onion (Green tops only)
Cabbage	Leek leaves	
Carrot	Butter lettuce	Squash (all except Butternut)
Celeriac	Radicchio lettuce	Swiss chard
Chicory leaves	Red Coral lettuce	Tomatoes
Chives	Olives	Turnip
Red Chili Pepper	Okra	Water chestnuts
Choy sum	Parsnip	Zucchini
Cucumber	Green pepper	Seaweed/Nori

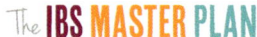

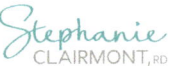

Moderate in FODMAPs	High in FODMAPs
Enjoy in small quantities	*Avoid these foods completely*
Canned artichoke hearts (⅛ cup)	Artichokes
Beetroot (½ medium)	Asparagus
Broccoli (½ cup)	Cauliflower
Butternut squash (¼ cup diced)	Garlic
Celery (¼ of a stalk)	Leeks
Savoy Cabbage (½ cup)	Mushrooms
Sweet corn (½ cobb)	Onions
Thawed green peas (¼ cup)	Shallots
Snow peas (5 pods)	Sugar snap peas
Sweet potato (½ cup)	
Sun-Dried tomatoes (1 Tbsp)	

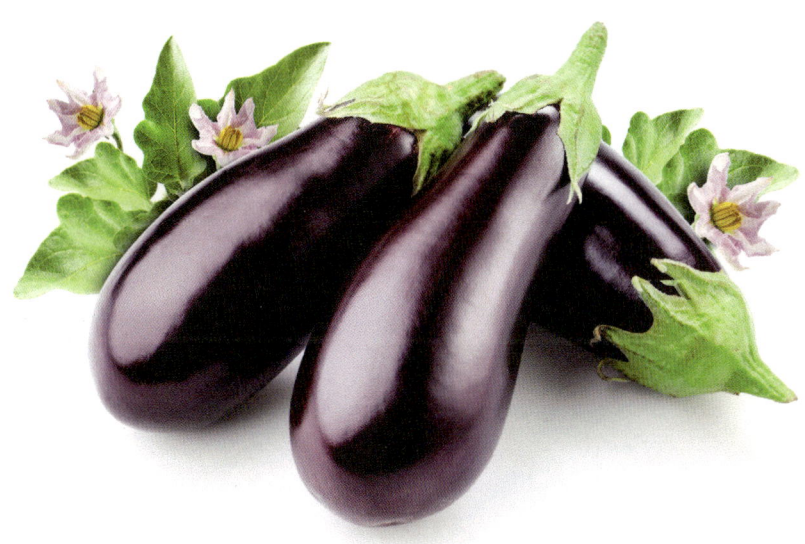

FRUIT

Fruit is full of amazing nutrients, fibre, is thirst-quenching, and a low calorie way to satisfy a sweet tooth. All fruit contains the sugar fructose, so even those that are low FODMAP fruit should be enjoyed in moderation. Enjoy several servings of fruit throughout the day at meals and/or snacks with one serving as approximately half a cup.

Low in FODMAPs

Include a variety of these foods every day, in servings of ½ cup at a time

Banana	Honeydew melon	Prickly pear
Blueberries	Kiwi	Pineapple
Cantaloupe melon	Lemon	Raspberries
Clementine	Lime	Rhubarb
Cranberries	Mandarin oranges	Star fruit
Dragon fruit	Navel oranges	Strawberries
Durian	Passion fruit	Tangelo
Grapes	Paw Paw	Tangerine

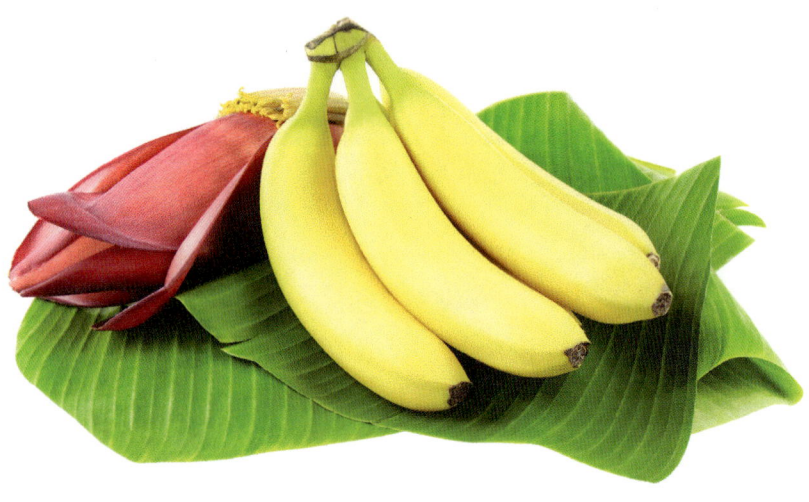

Moderate in FODMAPs	High in FODMAPs
Enjoy in small quantities	*Avoid these foods completely*
Dried banana (10 chips)	Apples
Coconut milk (½ cup)	Apricots
Dried, shredded coconut (¼ cup)	Blackberries
Dried cranberries (1 Tbsp)	Boysenberries
Currants (1 Tbsp)	Cherries
Grapefruit (½ medium)	Dried fruit (all including prunes and raisins)
Longon (5)	Figs
Lychee (5)	Mangoes
Pomegranate (¼ cup seeds)	Nectarines
	Peaches
	Pears (except Prickly variety)
	Persimmons
	Plums
	Tamarillo
	Watermelon

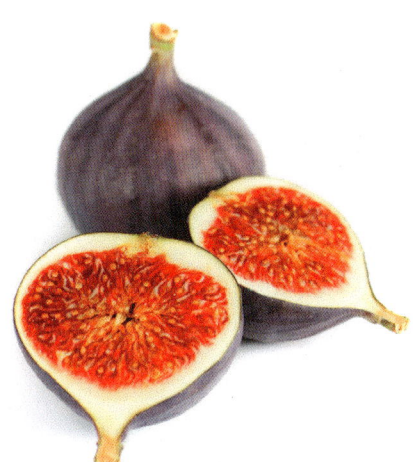

GRAINS & STARCHES

Carbohydrate foods get a bad rap in digestion as this group of food causes the most trouble. It's not necessary to cut out all carbohydrate foods which include cereals, grains, and starchy vegetables. These foods are the body's main source of energy, contain important nutrients, and help balance blood sugar. However, these foods require the most attention as many starchy products have a variety of ingredients. Check the ingredient list of foods like gluten free breads, crackers, and cereals to ensure they don't have other high FODMAP ingredients. Enjoy small portions of approximately ½ to 1 cup of grains and starches at each meal.

Low in FODMAPs

Include a variety of these foods every day; focus on unprocessed choices.

Arrowroot	Gluten-free cookies	Quinoa
Buckwheat	Gluten-free crackers	Quinoa flakes
Corn-based crackers	Gluten-free flour mixes	Quinoa pasta
Corn flour	Gluten-free pasta	Rice
Corn meal	Gluten-free soba noodles	Rice bran
Corn starch		Rice cakes, plain
Corn tortillas	Millet	Rice crackers
Gluten-free bread	Oat bran	Rice noodles
Gluten-free chia rice bread	Popcorn	Sorghum
	Potatoes	Spelt Sourdough Bread
Gluten-free multigrain bread	Potato chips	Tapioca
	Pretzels	

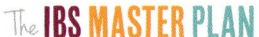
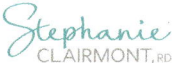

Moderate in FODMAPs

Some people may be able to enjoy small quantities (identified below) of the following foods after implementing the low FODMAP diet for several weeks. Be mindful of symptoms and listen to your body.

Amaranth, puffed (¼ cup)	Rice, puffed (½ cup)
Buckwheat kernels (⅛ cup)	Spelt pasta (½ cup)
Cornflakes Cereal (½ cup)	Wheat pasta (½ cup)
Oat Sourdough Bread (1 slice)	Wheat bran (½ tbsp)
Oats (¼ cup)	White or whole wheat bread (1 slice)

High in FODMAPs

Avoid these foods completely at the start of the low FODMAP diet. You may find you can tolerate these foods in small amounts later in the re-introduction phase of the diet.

Wheat-based products—bread, cereal, crackers, cookies, couscous, noodles, pasta

Rye-based products—bread, cereal, crackers, whole grains

Barley-based products—bread, cereal, crackers, whole grains

Inulin (derived from the chicory root)

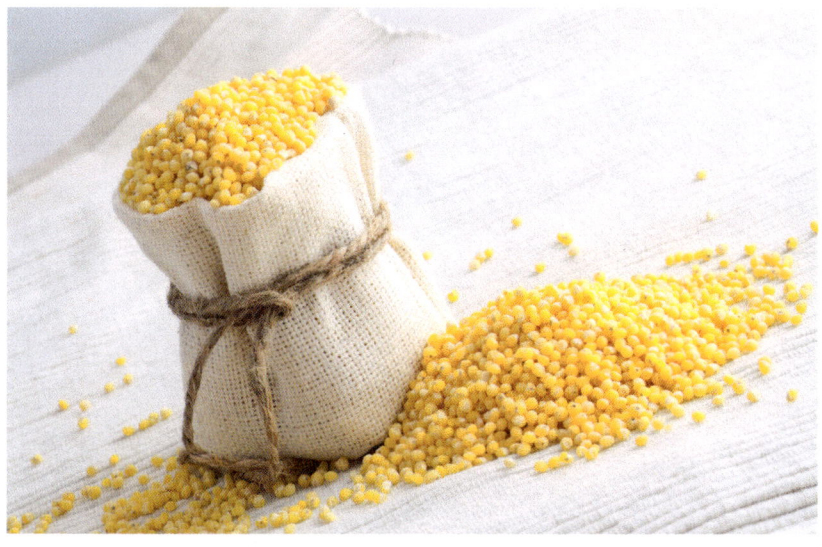

MEAT & ALTERNATIVES

The meat and alternative food group provides you with protein and is important to include several servings through the day at meals and snacks. If you are focusing on vegetarian proteins, include 4 or 5 servings daily. Although most meat products are low in FODMAPs, it is recommended to read food labels when purchasing packaged products like sausages and burgers to ensure there are not other high FODMAP or bothersome ingredients. Although low in FODMAPs, some individuals find high fat meals and red meat like beef and pork difficult on their digestion. Be mindful of your symptoms and listen to your body. Include healthy portions of approximately 2 ½ to 3 oz of meat, poultry, fish, tofu, or tempeh; ¼ cup lentils or chickpeas; 2 to 4 Tbsp nuts and seeds; or 2 eggs at each meal.

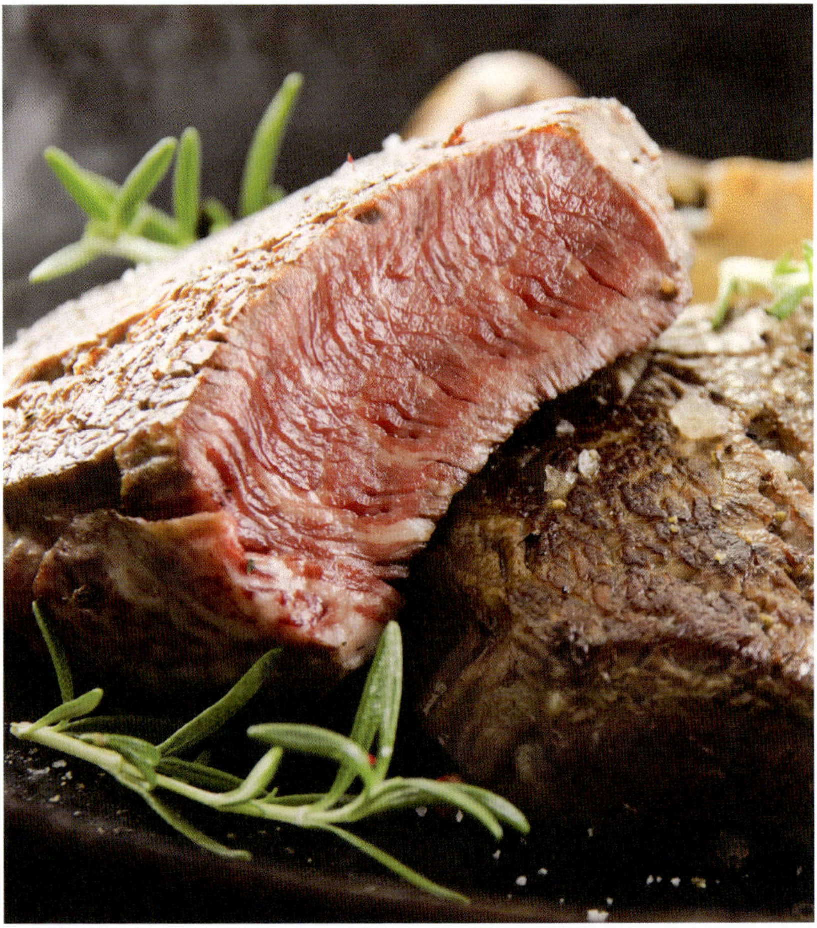

Low in FODMAPs

Include a variety of these foods every day.

Beef

Chicken

Eggs

Fish

Lamb

Pork

Tempeh

Tofu

Lentils, canned

Chia seeds

Macadamia nuts

Peanuts

Pecans

Pine nuts

Pumpkin seeds

Sesame seeds

Sunflower seeds

Walnuts

Moderate in FODMAPs

Enjoy in small quantities

Almonds (10 nuts)

Butter beans, canned (¼ cup)

Canned chickpeas (¼ cup)

Lentils, red or green, boiled (¼ cup)

Lima beans, boiled (¼ cup)

Hazelnuts (10 nuts)

High in FODMAPs

Avoid completely. Also, be cautious of meat products like burgers, chicken nuggets, and sausages to ensure they do not contain other FODMAP ingredients.

Baked beans

Borlotti beans

Broad beans

Four bean mix

Haricot beans, boiled

Red kidney beans

Soya beans, boiled

Split peas, boiled

Cashews

Pistachio

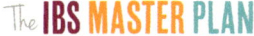
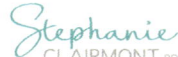

DAIRY & ALTERNATIVES

Dairy and alternative foods include milk, yogurt, and cheese made from Cow's, Goat's, or Sheep's milk as well as almond, soy, and rice. Not all foods in each of the categories have been tested yet for FODMAPs, so if the food is not listed on this page, no data existed at the time this book was released. It is important to note that although many dairy foods are low in FODMAPs, they may still cause digestive distress. You may need to consume the low FODMAP dairy foods in small quantities only. Every individual is different and has different triggers; work on being mindful of your body and the symptoms you experience to understand exactly what foods may contribute to your symptoms.

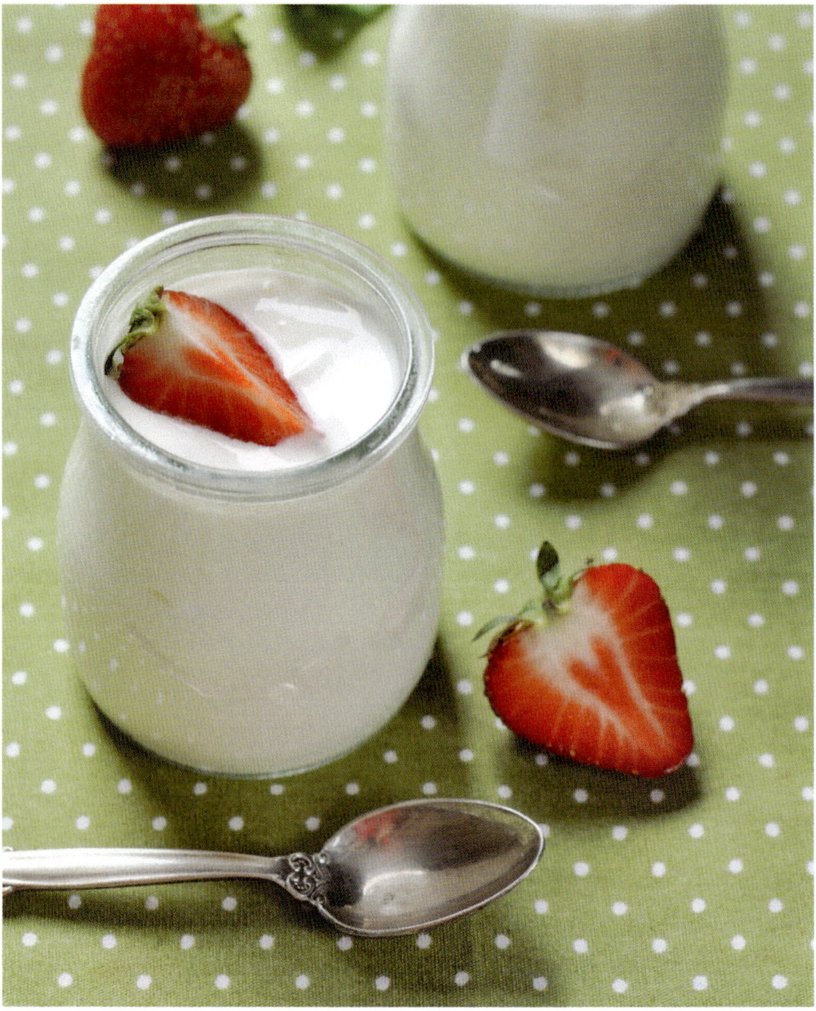

Low in FODMAPs

Enjoy a variety of these foods, but don't overindulge.

Brie cheese

Camembert cheese

Cheddar cheese

Colby cheese

Cottage cheese

Goat cheese

Feta cheese

Havarti cheese

Mozzarella cheese

Pecorino cheese

Swiss cheese

Lactose-free milk

Lactose-free yogurt

Coconut milk

Soy milk (made with soy protein)

Moderate in FODMAPs

Enjoy in small quantities

Haloumi cheese (2 slices)

Ricotta cheese (2 Tbsp)

Whipped cream (½ cup)

High in FODMAPs

Avoid completely

Buttermilk

Cream cheese

Cream, thickened, regular fat

Custard

Cow's milk (including homogenized, reduced fat, evaporated, skim, condensed)

Goat's Milk

Ice cream

Sour cream

Soy Milk (made with soy beans)

Yogurt (regular, low fat, flavoured)

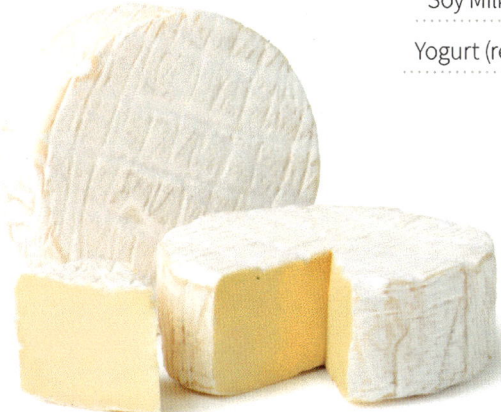

OTHER FOODS & INGREDIENTS

This category includes all foods that help to add flavour to your dish like herbs, spices, condiments, sauces, and spreads.

Low in FODMAPs

Include these in small amounts as desired

All Spice	Fats & Oils	Confectionaries
Basil	Olive Oil	Dark chocolate
Chives	Peanut Oil	<5 squares (30g)
Cilantro/Coriander	Rice Bran Oil	Milk chocolate <15 g
Cinnamon	Sesame Oil	White Chocolate <15 g
Cumin	Sunflower Oil	Stevia
Eggplant dip	Vegetable Oil	Brown Sugar
Five spice		Palm Sugar
Ginger root		Raw Sugar
Jam		White Sugar
Mustard		Maple Syrup
Peanut butter		Rice Malt Syrup
Paprika		
Parsley		
Rosemary		
Tarragon		
Thyme		
Tumeric		

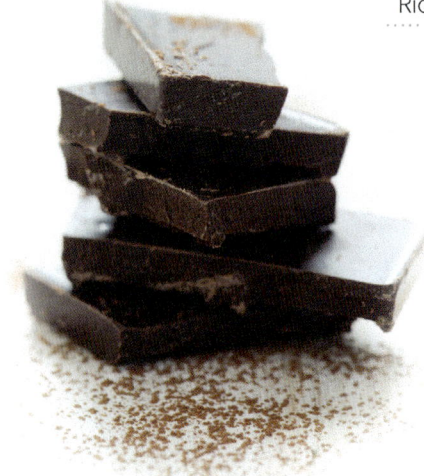

Moderate in FODMAPs

Enjoy these less often and in small quantities

Barbeque sauce (2 Tbsp)	**Beverages**
Balsamic vinegar (2 Tbsp)	Beer
Chutney (1 Tbsp)	Cranberry juice
Fish sauce (1 Tbsp)	Gin
Oyster sauce (1 Tbsp)	100% pure orange juice (½ cup)
Pesto sauce (1 Tbsp)	Vegetable juice (1 cup)
Pickled vegetables/relish (1 Tbsp)	Vodka
Rice Wine Vinegar (2 Tbsp)	Whisky
Soy sauce (2 Tbsp)	Wine (Red, White, Sweet, Sparkling)
Sweet and Sour sauce (2 Tbsp)	Hot Chocolate <2 tsp
Worcestershire sauce (2 Tbsp)	Vegetable blend tomato juice
Vegemite (1 tsp)	Instant regular & decaffeinated black coffee
	Espresso
	Tea (white, peppermint, green, dandelion)
	Herbal Tea (weak) <180 ml
	Chai Tea (weak) <180 ml
	Black Tea (strong) < 180 ml

High in FODMAPs

Avoid completely

Caviar Dip

Honey

Hummus

Jam – mixed berries

Ketchup

Tahini

Tzatziki dip

Pasta Sauce, cream-based

Pasta Sauce, tomato-based (pre-made)

Beverages

Apple juice

Cordial (apple, orange, raspberry)

Orange blended juice

Tropical and other juice blends

Rum

Wine, Sticky

Tea (oolong, fennel, chamomile)

Herbal Tea (strong)

Dandelion Tea (strong)

Chai Tea (strong)

Step 3: Get Your Fibre!

When following an exclusion diet that is gluten free and/or low in FODMAPs, it may seem like a challenge to get all the nutrients you need. Despite these food exclusions, there are still so many delicious, nutrient-packed foods that should be included. Fibre is one particular nutrient to be mindful of. A lack of fibre in your diet can result in loose stool and diarrhea, or slow digestion and constipation. Fibre makes a meal more satiating, balances blood sugars, helps lower cholesterol, and improves digestion. Fibre is not digestible; so including the right amount of fibre in the diet will help bulk up stool, reduce constipation and diarrhea, and aid in the movement of food and waste through your digestive tract. If your current way of eating is low in fibre, ensure you slowly increase your fibre intake and drink plenty of fluid throughout the day.

Here's what you need daily:

Women age 14 to 50:	25 g
Men age 14 to 50:	38 g
Women 51+:	21 g
Men 51+:	30 g

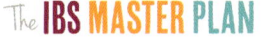
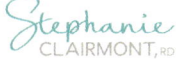

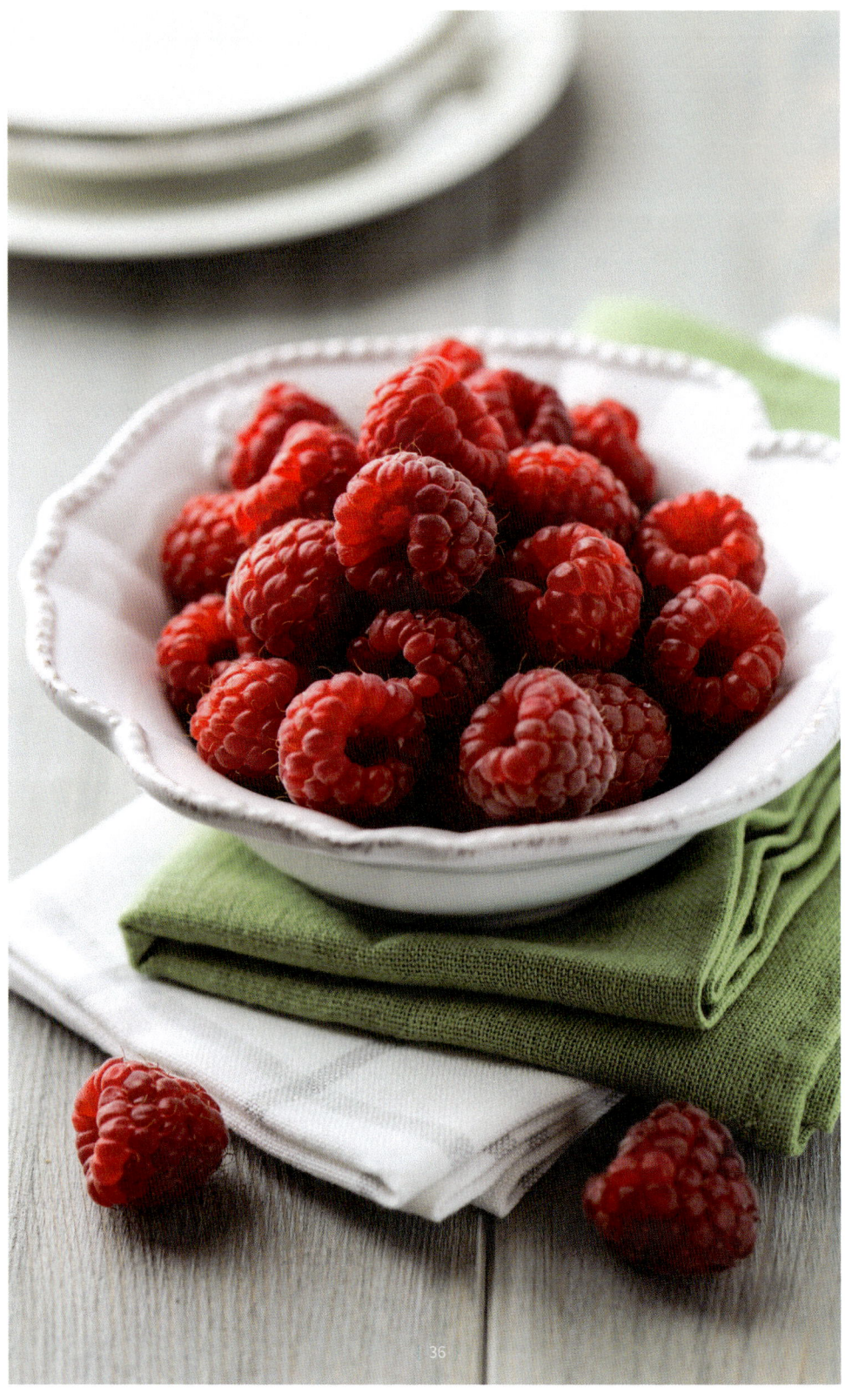

Top 5 Gluten Free, low FODMAP, Fibre-Rich foods:

1. **CHIA SEEDS: 12 GRAMS IN JUST 2 TBSP**
   Sprinkle on oatmeal, cereal, salads, stir-fry, fruit, or in baked goods

2. **OAT AND QUINOA FLAKES: 5 GRAMS IN A ½ CUP**
   Cook for breakfast, add to baked goods, or mix into smoothies

3. **RASPBERRIES: 4 GRAMS IN ½ CUP**
   Add to oatmeal, smoothies, or have as a snack

4. **SESAME SEED BUTTER: 4 GRAMS IN 2 TBSP**
   Add to homemade granola bars, shakes, or toast

5. **CANNED PUMPKIN: 4 GRAMS IN ½ CUP**
   Incorporate into healthy muffins, squares, bars, soups, or sauces

Find ways to include these foods every day to help you meet your fibre needs, or choose from the foods on the next page to add enough fibre-rich foods to keep your digestive system moving along.

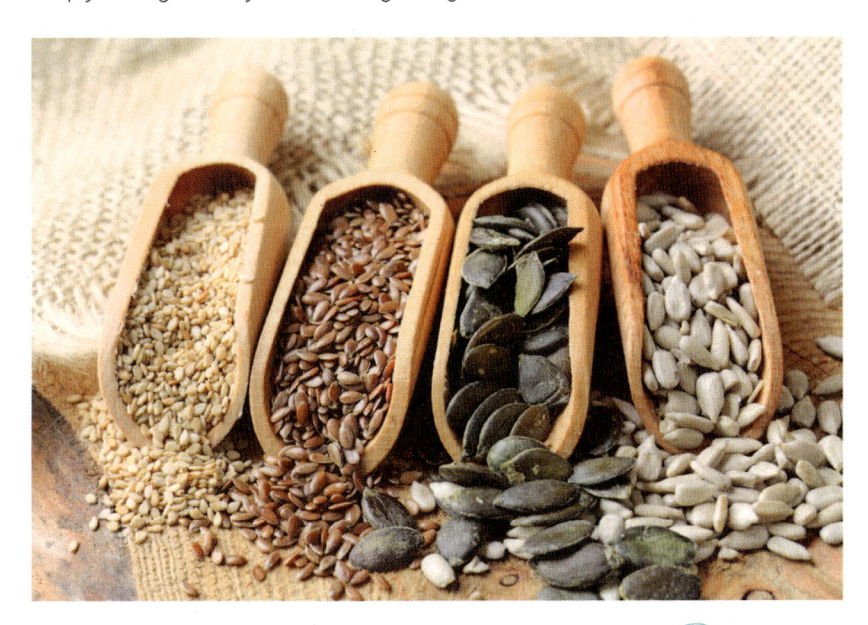

Fibre Content of Foods

SEEDS — ONE SERVING, ¼ CUP (4 TBSP)

Chia seeds	24 g
Ground flax seeds	6 g
Hemp seeds (hulled)	4 g
Sunflower seeds (hulled)	4 g
Sesame seeds	4 g
Pumpkin seeds	2 g

NUTS — ONE SERVING, ¼ CUP (4 TBSP)

Coconut, flesh, flaked	4 g
Peanuts	3 g
Walnuts	2 g
Pecans	2 g
Pine nuts	1 g

NUT BUTTERS — 2 TBSP

Sesame seed butter	4 g
Peanut butter	2 g

LEGUMES — ONE SERVING, ½ CUP COOKED OR CANNED, DRAINED

Lentils	6 to 8 g
Chickpeas	4 to 6 g

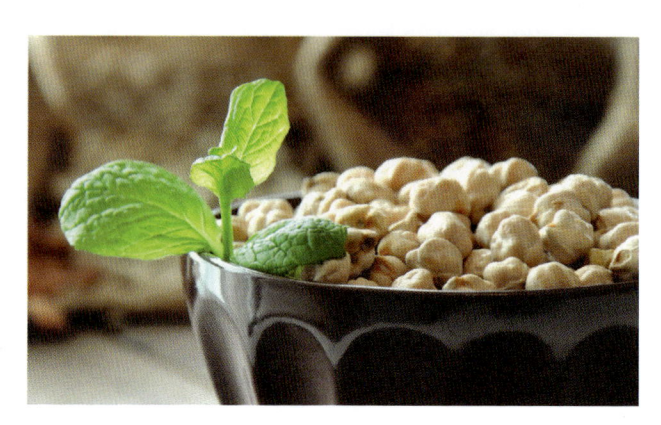

NOODLES — ONE SERVING:
35 TO 45 GRAMS, ABOUT ½ TO ¾ CUP COOKED

TruRoots Ancient grain pasta	3 g
Tinkyada brown rice pasta with rice bran	1 to 2 g
Tinkyada brown rice pasta	1 g
Corn pasta	0 to 1 g
Rice pasta	0 to 1 g
Soba noodles	0 to 1 g
Rice noodles	0 to 1 g

CEREALS — ½ CUP, RAW

Oats, large flake	5 g
Quinoa flakes	5 g

GRAINS — ¼ CUP, RAW

Millet	5 g
Quinoa	3 g
Wild rice blend (Lundberg)	3 g
Long grain brown rice (Lundberg)	3 g
Amaranth	3 g
White / sushi / Arborio rice	0 to 1 g

FLOURS & BRANS — ½ CUP

Rice bran (crude)	12 g
Stone ground whole grain corn flour (Bob's RM)	8 g
Oat bran	8 g
Almond flour	6 g
Whole grain oat flour	6 g
Quinoa flour	4 g
Brown rice flour	4 g
White rice flour	2 g
All-purpose GF blends	0 to 4 g

VEGETABLES

Potato, russet, white, or red	1 medium, baked	4 g
Pumpkin	½ cup, canned	4 g
Parsnip	½ cup, cooked	3 g
Squash, acorn, or butternut	½ cup, baked	2 g
Spinach	½ cup, cooked	2 g
Green beans	½ cup, cooked	2 g
Kale	½ cup, cooked	1.5 g
Zucchini	½ cup, cooked	1.5 g
Eggplant	½ cup, cooked	1.5 g
Fennel	½ cup, raw	1.5 g
Red bell pepper	½ cup, cooked	1.5 g
Turnip	½ cup, cooked	1.5 g
Spinach	1 cup, raw	1 g
Bell pepper	½ of a raw pepper	1 g
Bean sprouts	½ cup, cooked	1 g
Broccoli	½ cup, raw	1 g
Bok Choy	½ cup, cooked	1 g
Cabbage, red or green	½ cup, raw	1 g
Carrots	½ cup, cooked	1 g
Tomato	½ cup, canned or raw	1 g
Arugula	1 cup, raw	0.5 g
Yellow bell pepper	½ cup, cooked	0.5 g

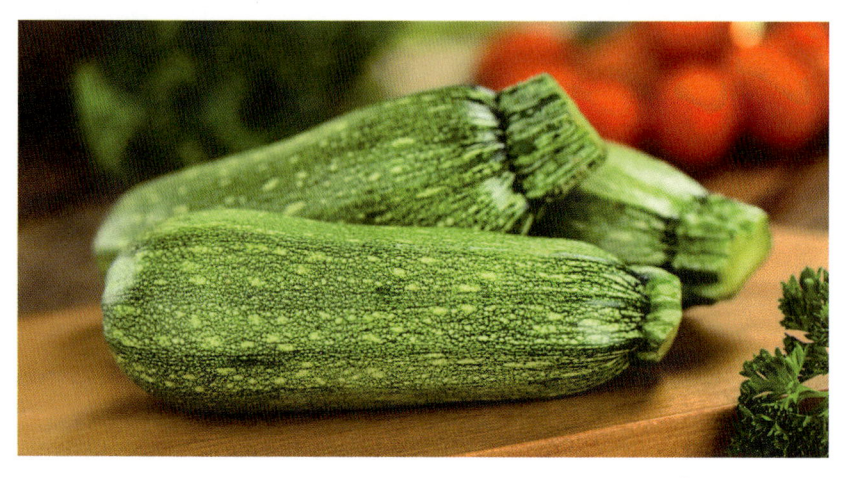

FRUIT — 1 SERVING

Raspberries	1 cup	8 g
Kiwi fruit	2	5 g
Blueberries	1 cup	4 g
Strawberries	1 cup	3 g
Orange, navel	1	3 g
Rhubarb	½ cup, cooked	2.5 g
Banana	1 medium	2 g
Clementine	1	1.5 g
Mandarin	1 medium	1.5 g
Pineapple	½ cup	1 g
Grapes	½ cup	0.5 g
Melon, cantaloupe or honeydew	½ cup	0.5 g

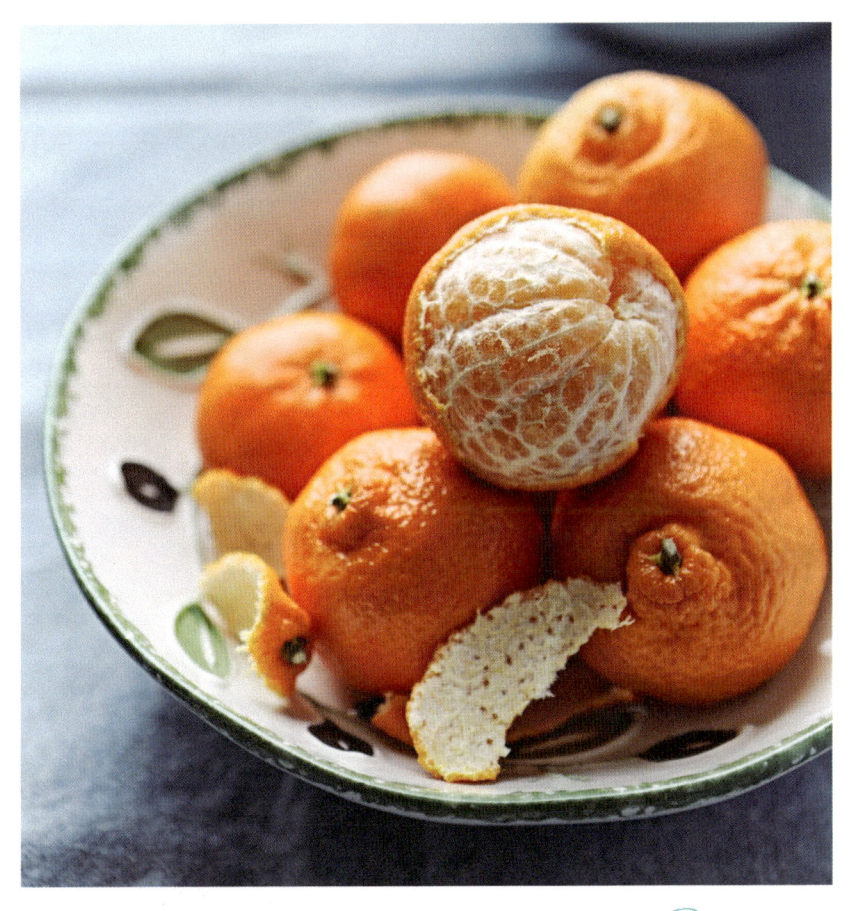

Step 4:
Make Every Day a Healthy Eating Day

While excluding the foods that may be causing digestive distress, it's important to continue to eat well. What does healthy eating mean? It means getting all the foods you need to ensure you get enough vitamins, minerals, and nutrients to keep your body working well. Stick to real, wholesome food and limit packaged food. Here is an outline of how to create balanced meals and snacks throughout the day. This is a general overview for one day. Depending on your age, height, weight, and activity level, you may need more or less at each meal. You may not need three snacks each day either. It is recommended you work with a *registered dietitian* to decide what the best schedule of eating is for you.

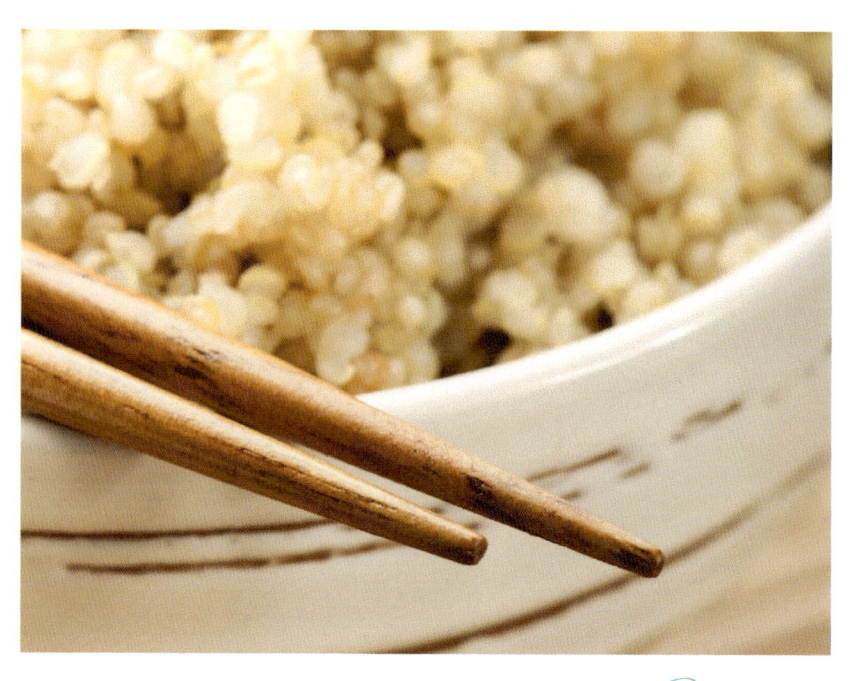

Healthy Eating One Day Formula

MEAL	WHAT TO EAT
Breakfast	1 cup cooked oatmeal OR 1 cup cooked potato OR 2 slices Udi's white toast (or other low FODMAP bread) OR 2 servings other low FODMAP grain/starch + one serving of protein such as 1 to 2 eggs OR 2 oz fish/poultry/meat OR 2 Tbsp nuts/seeds/nut butters OR ½ cup LF yogurt OR ¼ cup cottage cheese
Snack	½ cup of low FODMAP fruit + half (to one) serving of protein such as 1 to 2 Tbsp nuts/seeds/nut butters OR 1 oz cheese OR ¼ to ½ cup LF yogurt or cottage cheese
Lunch	½ to 1 cup of grains & starches such as wild/brown/white rice, corn pasta, rice noodle, potato, squash, quinoa, or millet OR 1 to 2 slices of low FODMAP bread + 1 ½ to 2 cups of low FODMAP vegetables + protein such as 3 oz lean meat/poultry/fish/seafood/tofu/tempeh OR 2 eggs OR ¼ cup lentils OR a combination of these ingredients
Snack	½ cup of low FODMAP fruit + half (to one) serving of protein such as 1 Tbsp nuts/seeds/nut butters OR 1 oz cheese OR ¼ cup LF yogurt or cottage cheese
Dinner	½ to 1 cup of grains & starches OR 1 to 2 slices of low FODMAP bread + 1 ½ to 2 cups of vegetables + protein (as outlined above in lunch)
Snack	(If needed; i.e., after exercise, staying up late, or if having an early dinner, etc.) ½ cup of low FODMAP fruit AND/OR handful of nuts AND/OR ¼ to ½ cup LF yogurt or cottage cheese OR a homemade smoothie

NOTE FROM THE KITCHEN:

Choose lean protein more often, include fish 2 to 4 times per week, enjoy vegetarian meals several times per week including lentils, tofu, or tempeh.

Step 5: Make a Plan for Success

When you're trying to follow a diet different than what you are used to, there are a lot of changes to be made. This can be extremely overwhelming, unless you make a plan and stick to it. Meal planning will save you time and money, plus having a plan will help you feel in control and reduce stress significantly. Here's what to do:

1. CHOOSE YOUR RECIPES

Do some foodie research! Visit blogs, use your favourite cookbooks, check out some gluten free or health food magazines, and follow some low FODMAP Pinterest boards to find delicious recipes that appeal to you. There are several resources for low FODMAP recipes, but you can also look up gluten free, dairy-free recipes and just change a few ingredients to avoid foods that are symptom triggers for you. Here are a few recommended sources, recipes from any of these websites would be beneficial:

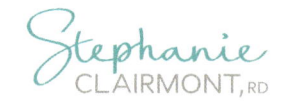

Stephanie Clairmont, RD

www.stephanieclairmont.com

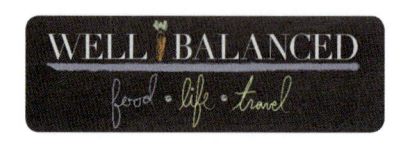

WELL BALANCED — food • life • travel

http://blog.katescarlata.com

Low FODMAP.com

http://www.lowfodmap.com

2. CREATE AN ACTUAL MEAL PLAN

Write out the days of the week on a chalk or white board in your kitchen, use the Make-Your-Own-Meal Plan Tool, or use the meal plan template on the next page. Use the recipes you've chosen for the week to plan evening meals only or both lunch and dinner and fit them into the template to identify what meals you would like on what days. Try to space out meat, fish, and vegetarian meals so that you are planning a variety of proteins for health. When possible, consider making big batches to use leftovers for lunch or busy nights of the week. Choose local, seasonal foods as much as possible. Consider using the meal plans available in Chapter Three of this book.

3. MAKE A SHOPPING LIST

Create categories according to sections in your grocery store like produce, breads & grains, meats, fish & other proteins, and fridge/freezer section. Write down according to your plan what you need from each section.

4. GET YOUR GOODS

Visit your local market, shop at farm stores, and choose local, seasonal, and organic or naturally raised as often as possible. Don't forget to assess what you have already at home and exclude it from your list. Stick to your list to avoid buying things you don't need and stay on budget. Shop the perimeter of the grocery store where you will find the healthiest food. It's important to not stock up on boxed and packaged food, even if it fits within the guidelines—focus on real, wholesome food for health.

Tip:

Get everyone in the family involved in planning and cooking to make the experience more enjoyable, save time in the kitchen, and ensure there are no complaints!

Weekly Meal Planner	Groceries Needed:
M	
T	
W	
T	
F	
S	
S	

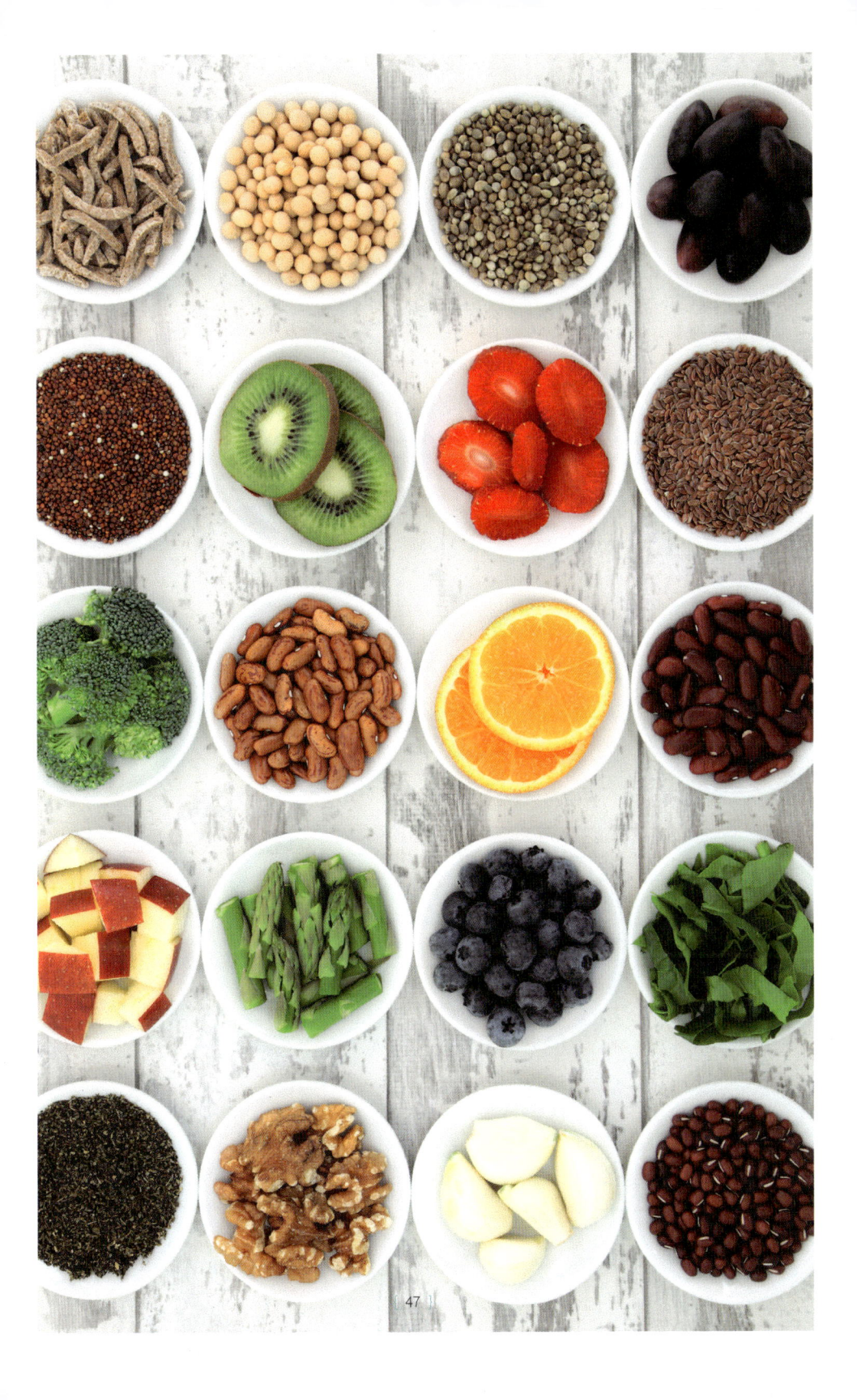

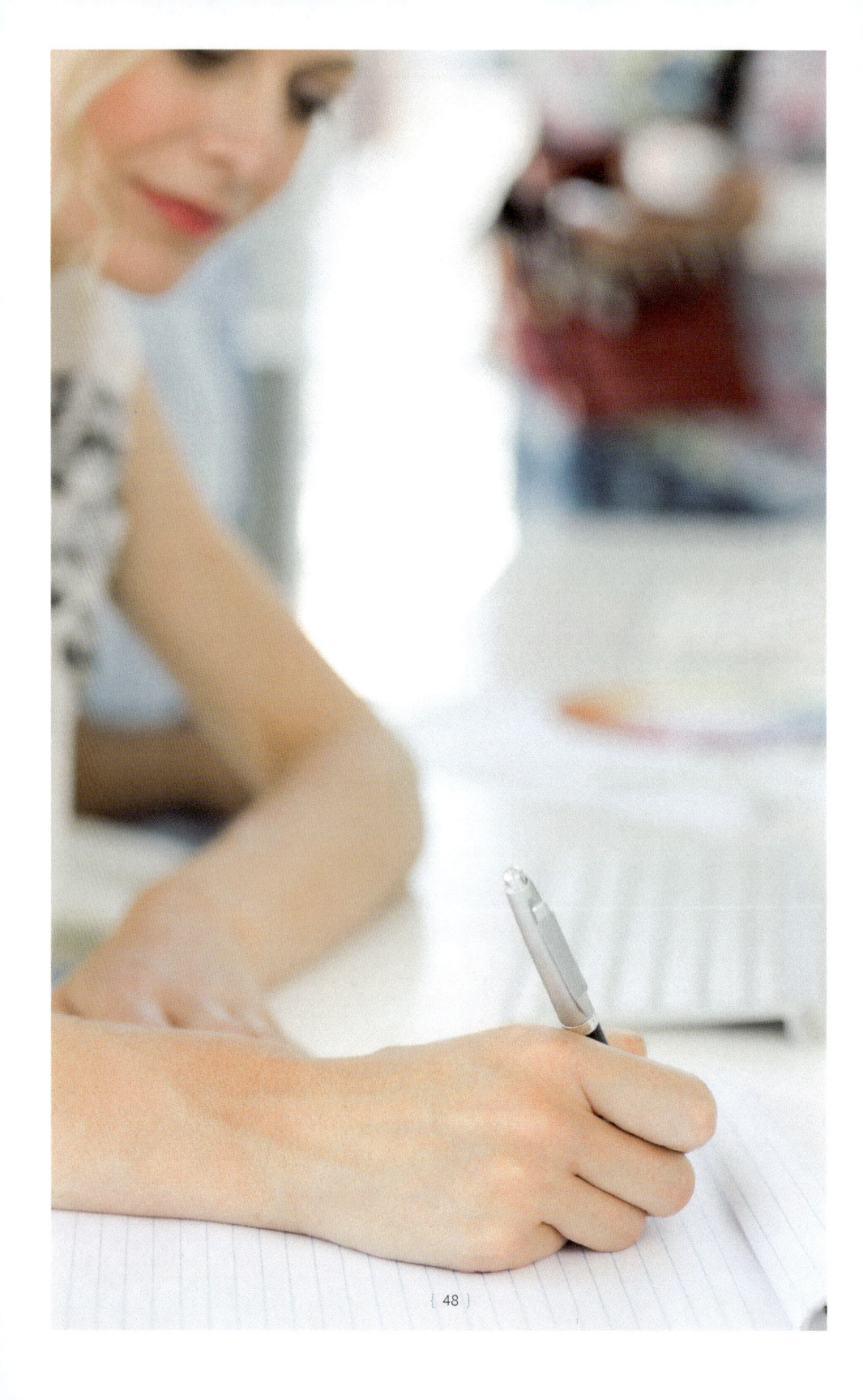

Step 6:
Keep a Food & Symptom Journal

When you experience digestive symptoms such as gas, bloating, abdominal distention, pain, diarrhea, and constipation—it can be frustrating and embarrasing. The most effective way to get through this, especially while making changes to your diet is by keeping a journal. Use the template on the next page by either transferring it into a notebook, printing multiple copies, or copying into a word or excel file. Start by tracking your intake for one week before you make changes to assess what your symptoms are from the start. Keep track of your intake and symptoms for the 2 to 4 months you implement the IBS Master Plan and keep tracking when starting the reintroduction phase. You must stay committed to recording—it's the key to helping you identify your personal triggers and tracking improvement. This journal will become a tool you can review with your doctor and/or registered dietitian. By working with a dietitian, especially one that specializes in digestive nutrition, you will get expert advice on identifying symptom patterns, ensure you are doing everything needed to get better, and help you identify triggers that you may be missing.

In addition to documenting food patterns, begin to engage your mind by completing regular body scans. Notice stress and tension in your body and observe how stress, tension, or anxiety may be influencing your food patterns. Consult a registered social worker or other mental health specialist to ensure you are integrating the mind-body approach into your daily plan.

How to Keep a Food and Symptom Journal

Consider tracking multiple factors.
In your journalling include:

- Exactly what you eat and drink, including brand names and amounts (don't forget condiments, sauces, and seasonings)

- The order that you eat food in (some foods are ok on a full stomach but not empty)

- When you eat

- Where you are when you eat

- How you feel—is it a hectic morning grab & go breakfast, lunch at your desk while working, or a relaxing candle lit dinner?

- What symptoms you feel and rate the severity from 1 to 10—include everything from gas and bloating to headaches and energy levels

- When you have a bowel movement (BM) and what type according to the Bristol Stool Chart numbering system

- Complete Body Scan for the day. Is there tension in your body? Document where you are feeling this tension.

- List if the following triggers were present at all during the day, what they were, and when you felt them:

  1. Environment (i.e. bad weather, rainy day)
  2. People
  3. Events
  4. Situations (i.e. child is sick, conflict with a co-worker, etc.)

- Make a plan for self-care. What do you plan on doing to decrease tension, stress, or anxiety? Consult the Tips for Tips for Taking Emotional Breaks handout for suggestions on page 63.

BRISTOL STOOL CHART

Type 1		Separate hard lumps, like nuts (hard to pass)
Type 2		Sausage-shaped but lumpy
Type 3		Like a sausage but with cracks on the surface
Type 4		Like a sausage or snake, smooth and soft
Type 5		Soft blobs with clear-cut edges
Type 6		Fluffy pieces with ragged edges, a mushy stool
Type 7		Watery, no solid pieces. Entirely Liquid

Bristol Stool chart original source: Lewis SJ, Heaton KW (1997). *"Stool form scale as a useful guide to intestinal transit time".* Scand. J. Gastroenterol. 32 (9): 9204.

Food and Symptom Journal

Keep record of your intake, symptoms, and plan of care for 2 to 4 months while making changes.

Name:

Date:

Time of Day/Meal *i.e. breakfast, snack, etc.*	Intake	Situational Triggers *i.e. environment, people, eating in a hurry etc.*	Symptoms *(conduct body scan for tension and anxiety) i.e. gas, bloating, pain, anxiety, etc.*	Bowel *Movements— number and Type (Use Bristol Stool Chart)*	Plan for Self-Care *(use tips from "Taking Emotion Breaks" section)*

Additional Notes:

The IBS MASTER PLAN

Stephanie CLAIRMONT, RD

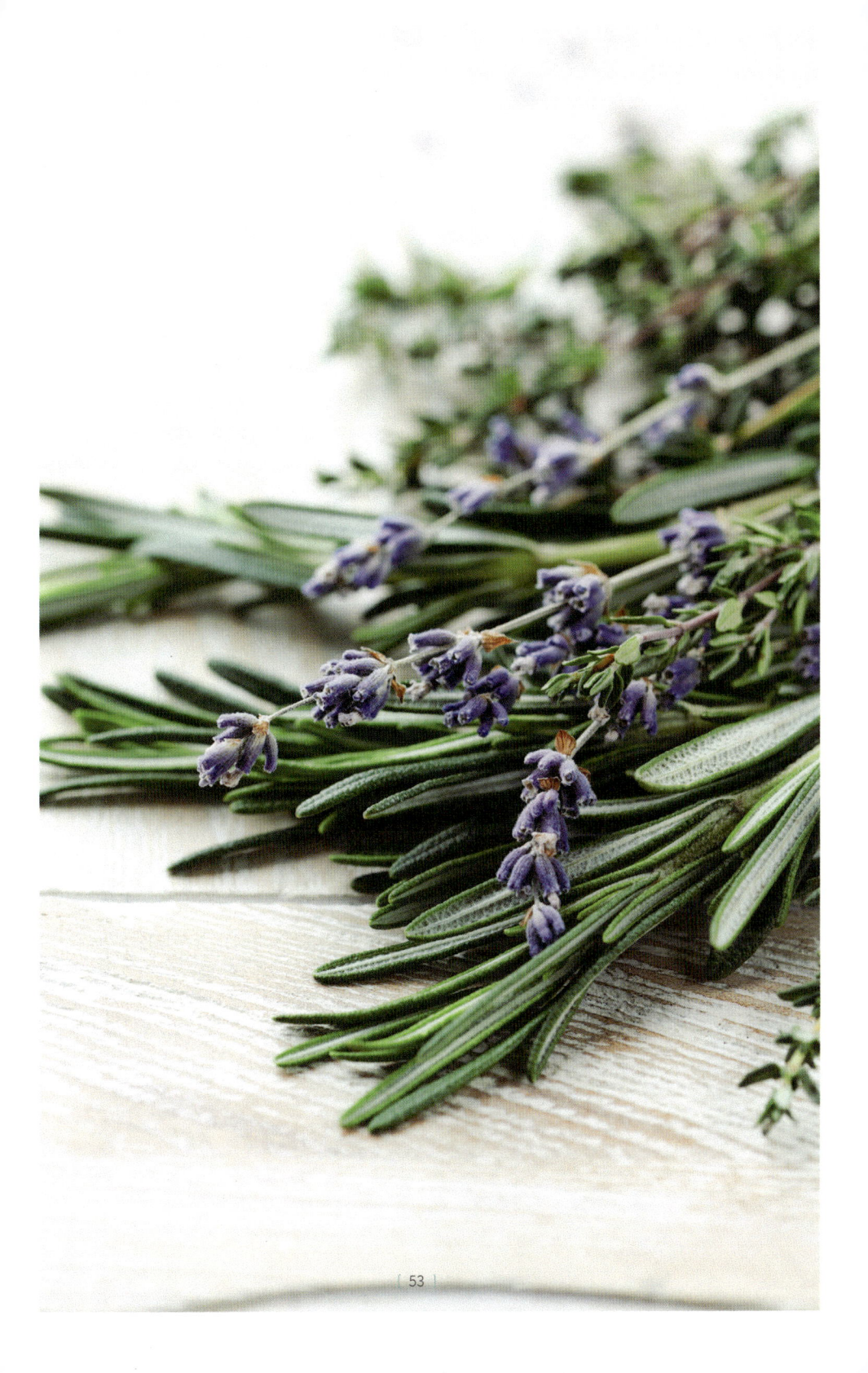

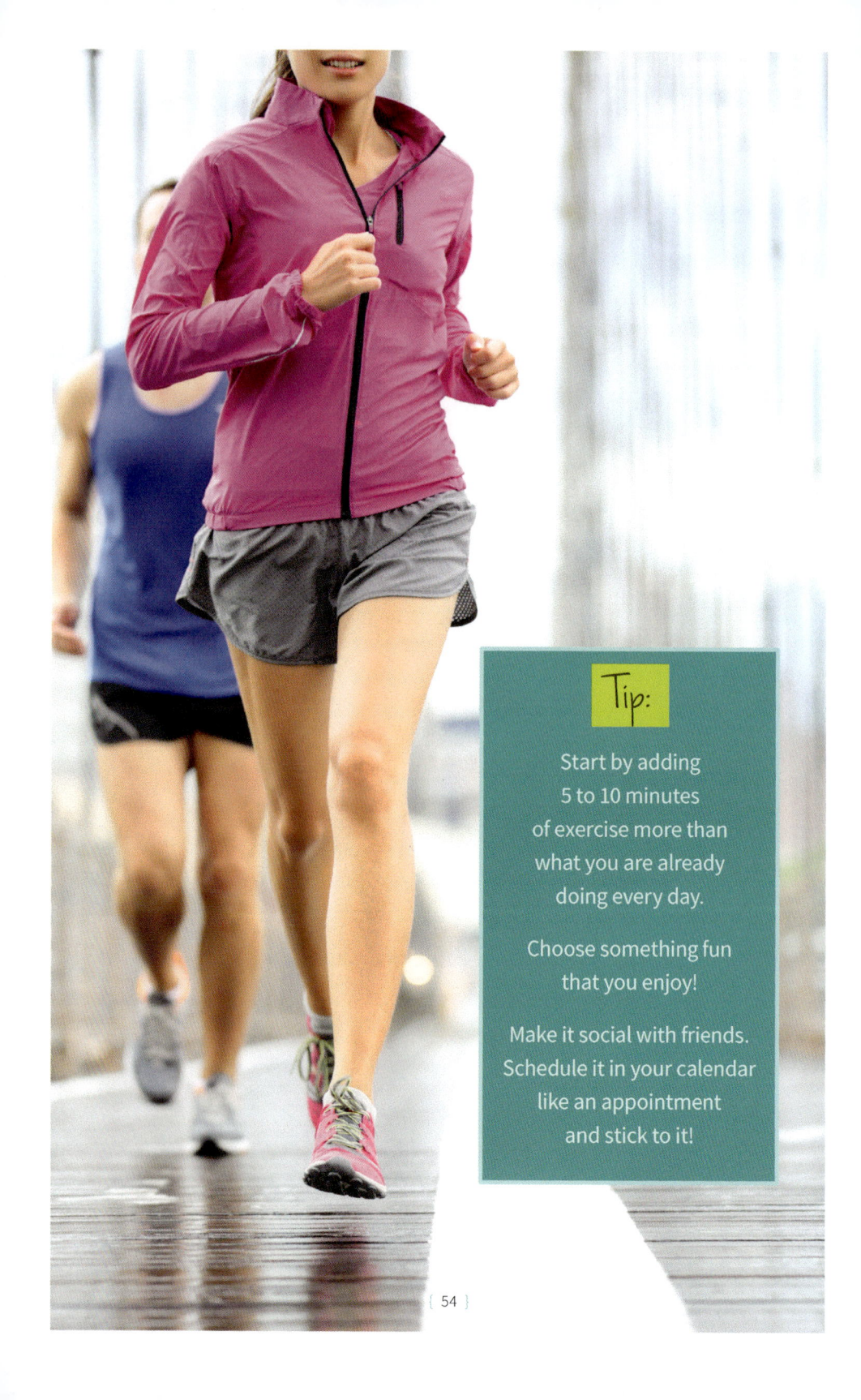

Tip:

Start by adding
5 to 10 minutes
of exercise more than
what you are already
doing every day.

Choose something fun
that you enjoy!

Make it social with friends.
Schedule it in your calendar
like an appointment
and stick to it!

Step 7:
Be Active Every Day

You may wonder what exercise has to do with IBS. Well, we know exercise has many benefits from helping us reach or maintain a healthy weight, to lowering risk of heart disease and cancer, to improving flexibility and strength. Regular activity helps your body to function the best it can, so it directly relates to how your digestive system works. In addition to this, exercise helps to reduce stress. Stress and anxiety are one of the major triggers for symptoms of IBS and digestive distress. Most clients of the Clairmont Digestive Clinic can directly relate stressful days or events to an increase in symptoms. If you cannot make this connection, challenge yourself to increase your awareness of how you feel daily. Consult your Food & Symptom Journal to observe any patterns of stress, anxiety, or tension throughout the week. Step 8 will discuss the mind-body connection further.

During exercise, our bodies release endorphins, the "feel-good" hormones that help us naturally feel good. Exercise can provide an escape to bothersome thoughts and issues that can crowd our day, gives us a break from the stresses of work, school, and life, and can be an outlet for aggressive or negative impulses.

To increase your activity, the first thing is to create a new habit. This is one of the most challenging things you will ever experience. Breaking and developing habits requires behaviour change and boy is that difficult! Look at your day and your week and figure out the best time for you to include exercise. You need to plan for success. Make it easy on yourself by choosing activities or partners that you enjoy or so that you'll look forward to exercise in your day.

HERE ARE SOME SIMPLE SUGGESTIONS TO GET YOU STARTED:

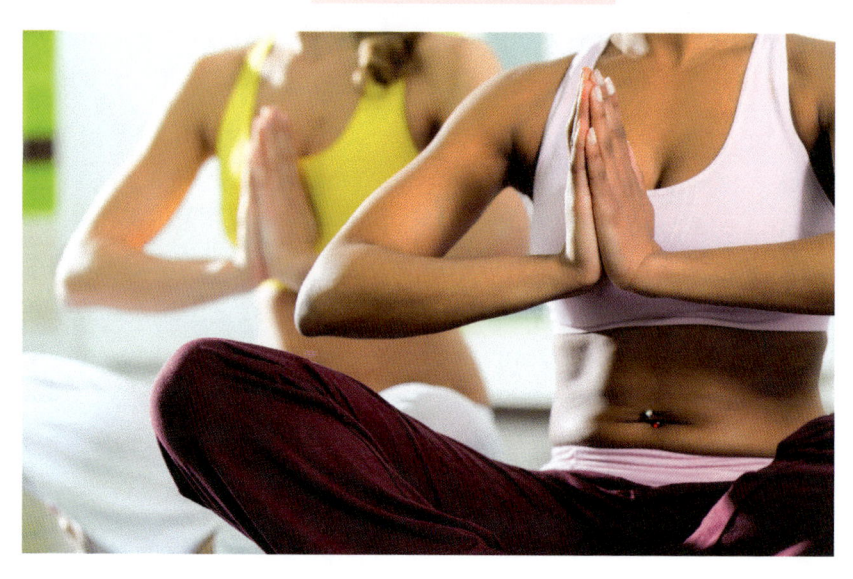

- Park further away from work to get a morning and evening walk of 5 to 10 minutes in every day.
- Consider riding your bike to work in warm weather
- Take a walk after lunch and dinner. NOTE: this can also faciliate gut motility and help you digest your food better
- Take a morning or afternoon break from work. Get up and go for a walk.
- Schedule stretching or yoga breaks for 5 to 10 minutes, several times during your day.
- Get a mini trampoline or skipping rope for your home or office and jump for 5 minutes a couple times during the day or on commercial breaks when watching tv.
- Join a fun class with a friend like Zumba, dancing, water aerobics, kickboxing, or whatever you enjoy.
- Schedule walks with friends and family instead of meeting for coffee or lunch.
- Organize group acitivites on the weekend that involve exercise like mini-putting, frisbee golf, bocce (lawn bowling), or another sport you enjoy.
- Consult the Tips for Taking Emotional Breaks handout for more ideas

Step 8: Work on Mind-Body Balance

by Bina Moore, MSW

As mentioned before, our mind and body are completely related. Stress and anxiety can be huge triggers to digestive distress. Many of the clients at the Clairmont Digestive Health Clinic are supported by our Digestive Health Therapist. These clients are often shocked to hear of the correlation between Anxiety and Irritable Bowel Syndrome (IBS). What is Anxiety? Excellent question! Anxiety is the body's way of responding to being in danger.

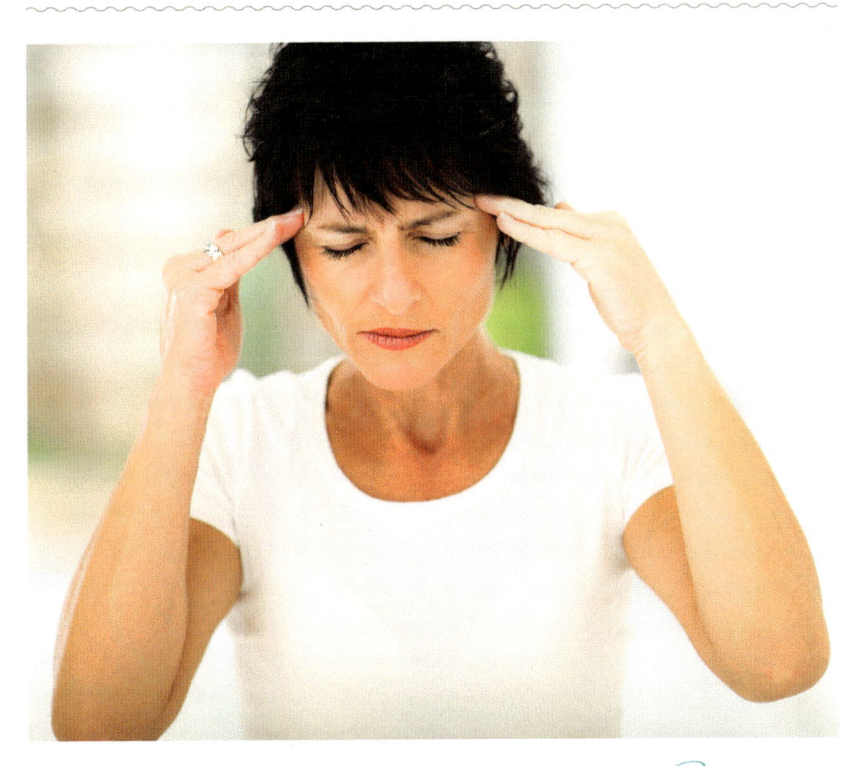

TRAUMA/ STRESS/ANXIETY
↓
FIGHT/FLIGHT/FREEZE RESPONSE
↓
RELEASE OF STRESS HORMONE OR BODY RESPONSES

Adrenaline is rushed into our bloodstream to enable us to run away or fight. This happens whether the danger is real, or whether we believe the danger is there when actually there is none. It is the body's alarm and survival mechanism. Primitive man wouldn't have survived for long without this life-saving response! Our brain has now registered the feeling of 'fear' allowing for possible anxiety episodes regardless if there is perceived danger or not.

Symptoms of Anxiety can have a very **intense effect** on your body chemistry occasionally changing your hormone production, altering your immune system, and in some cases, upsetting your digestive tract. Anxiety has been linked to contributing the development of IBS, also known as spastic colon- a chronic condition that includes bloating, gastrointestinal discomforts, erratic bowel movements, chronic abdominal pain, diarrhea, and constipation. If you are unsure that you are experiencing anxiety, here are a few physical sensations that will trigger an adrenaline response in your body:

- Fast-paced breathing
- Dizzy or light headed
- Muscle tensions
- Sweating
- Fast heart beat
- Chronic headaches, back and neck tension
- Persistent fatigue
- High blood pressure
- Irritability
- Overwhelming anxiety
- Sleep disturbances
- Digestive health issues (flare up)

Behaviours might include:

- Avoiding people or places
- Going to certain places at certain times, leaving early
- Coping behaviours; i.e., smoking, drinking, fiddling, increasingly talkative, quiet or withdrawn, avoiding eye contact, etc.
- Conflict

The Mind/Body Approach

Gabor Maté is one of the leading researchers in this field of study. His latest work focuses on how stress impacts the body. In his book, *When the Body Says No: The Hidden Costs of Stress,* he argues that due to busyness of day-to-day life we do not pay enough attention to what or bodies are telling us. We become so overwhelmed with day-to-day tasks that we fail to engage in daily self-care.

The Mind-body approach, through a variety of techniques and practices **enhances** body & symptom awareness. This approach can be helpful for any individual, practice, or profession. In our practice we have seen this be particularly important for individuals struggling with Digestive Health Issues because they first and foremost become more aware of stress and tension within their body. Techniques and strategies encourage relaxation, improve coping skills, reduce tension and pain, support and reduce anxiety and depression, and in some cases lessen the need for medication.

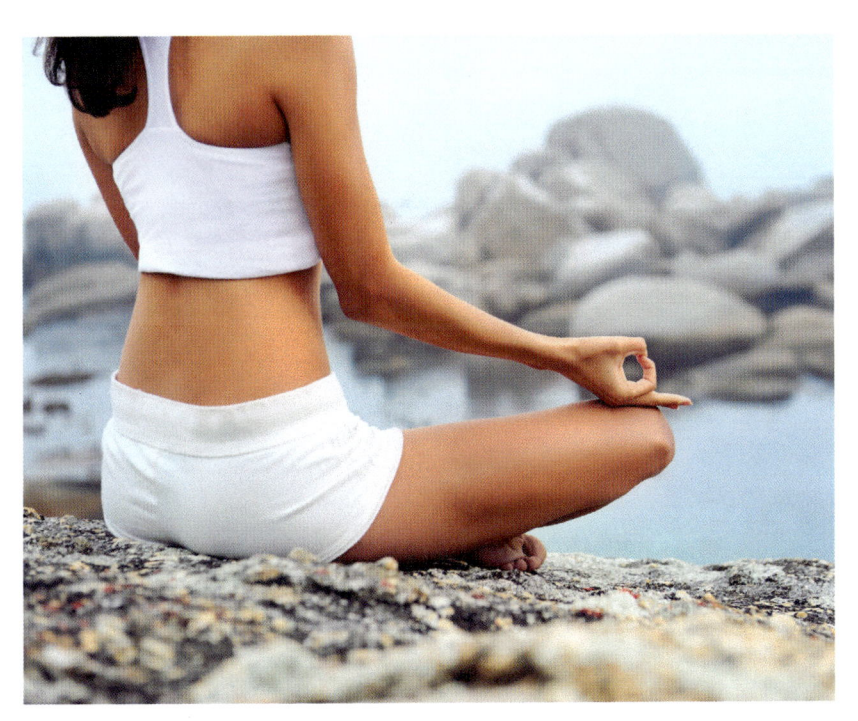

Here are 3 Strategies to help you get started with your Mind/Body Awareness

1. TENSE-AND-RELEASE PROGRESSIVE MUSCLE RELAXATION

Progressive muscle relaxation for tension release is a "first line" treatment for the physical tension of the anxious body. When combined with slow, deep breathing, this intentional relaxation of muscles helps the parasympathetic nervous system lower blood pressure and slow heart rate and respiration. This technique not only eliminates tension-related stiffness and aches but also lowers arousal levels, which makes triggering anxious physical symptoms more difficult.

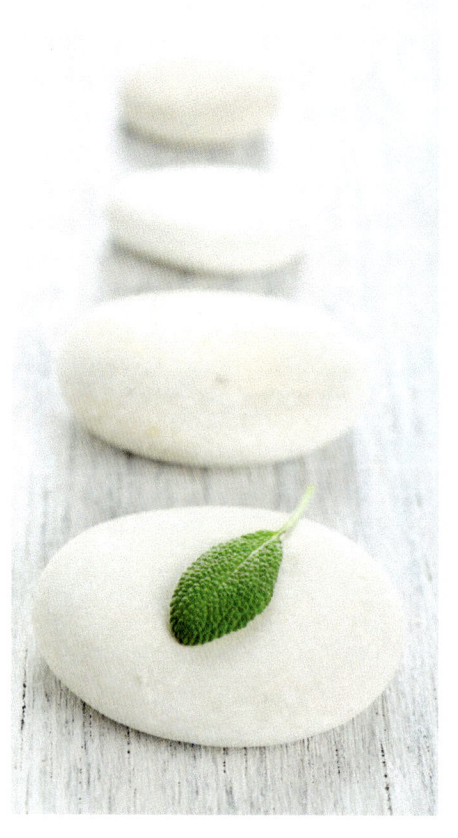

- Tighten and release each muscle group-slowly progressing from head to toes.

- Follow this order: head, neck, shoulders, arms, hands/fingers, chest, abdomen, hips, thighs, shins/calves, ankles, feet, and toes.

- Before moving from one group to the next notice your breathing. Breathe in through your nose and out through your mouth.

- End with noticing how calm your body is feeling. If you are feeling positive, recite a positive affirmation. Example: "I am a good person" or "I will get through this stress". Continue for 3 breaths before opening your eyes, and bringing your awareness back to the room.

2. SIMPLE BREATHING TECHNIQUES

Paying attention to your breathing is one of the most fundamental ways to relieve anxiety and tension. Here are a couple of simple ways to improve your breathing when you begin to notice stress, tension, or anxiety within your body.

Diaphragmatic Breathing

Begin by placing one hand on your stomach and the other one on your chest, and observe which one rises as you breathe in. If you notice your chest rising, it may mean you are breathing too shallowly (most of us do). This type of breathing may contribute to an increase in anxiety and tension. When we engage in 'Deep Breathing' we breathe into our diaphragm, a dome-shaped muscle, which expands allowing our stomach to rise as we breathe into it.

- Imagine that you have a bowl in your stomach that you are trying to fill in with air.
- See that stream of clean fresh air going down all the way into your stomach to fill the "bowl".
- Practice breathing deeper until you can get your stomach to rise consistently on in-breath.

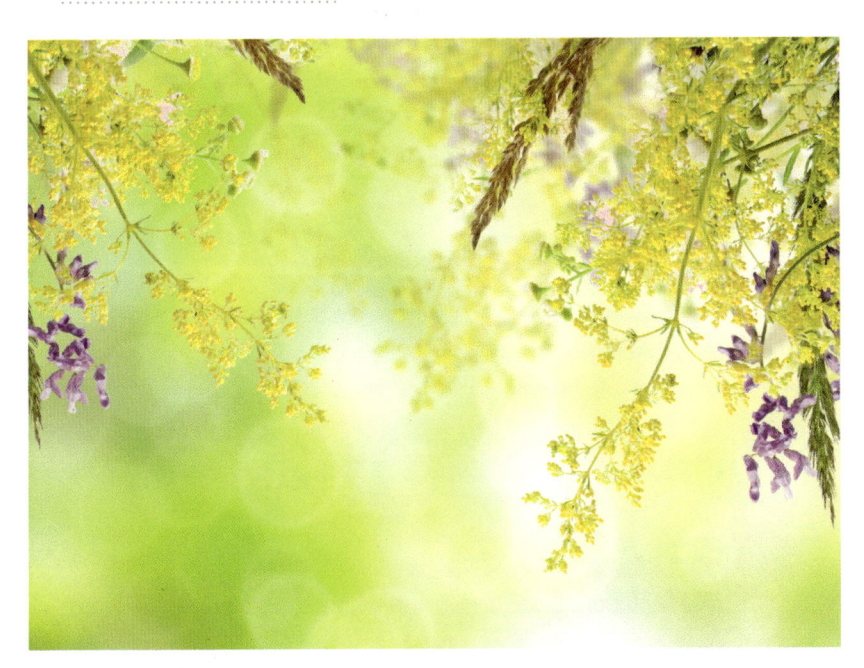

Square Breathing

"Square breathing" is a simple breathing technique that can be completed in any environment. Follow these 4 simple instructions:

1. Breathe in as you count to 4
2. Hold your breath to the count of 4
3. Breath out to the count of 4
4. Count to 4 before breathing in again.

It can be helpful to rest your eyes on each side of a square for the steps 1–4 as you perform this exercise. Repeat a number of times.

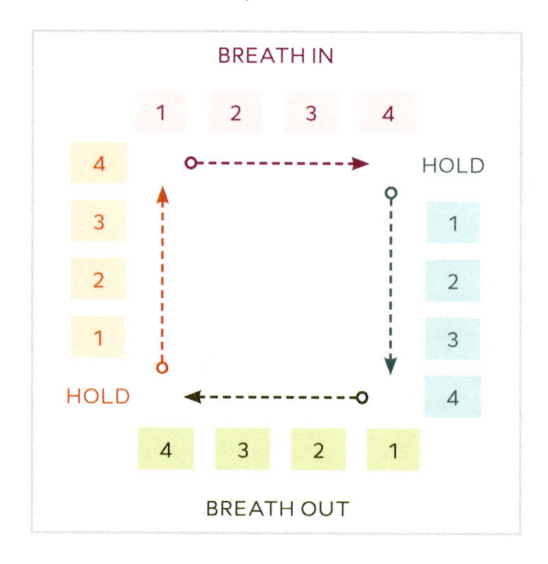

Yogi Breathing

To engage yourself in Yogi breathing find a place in your home or a spot in your office where you feel comfortable sitting in an upright position. When you are ready, place your right pointer finger on your right nostril. Breathe in through your left nostril then remove your right index finger from your right nostril, place your left pointer finger on your left nostril and breathe out through your right nostril. Continue alternating as you only breathe through one nostril at a time. This breathing technique will increase the oxygen to your brain in addition to reducing tension within the body.

3. TIPS FOR TAKING EMOTIONAL BREAKS

Taking emotional breaks every 2–3 hours throughout your day ensures you incorporating self-care activities that can support the release of tension or anxiety from your body. Due to the business of work, personal life, family, etc. we often forget to 'carve out' time from our day that is dedicated to increasing our mind/body awareness. Take out your daily planners and outline time even if it is only 5 minutes for self-care activities. Our 'Tips for taking Emotional Breaks' may provide you with a few ideas to get you started.

1. Change what is happening with your senses in the moment.

   › **Sight:** read a book or magazine, watch a funny show, take a walk

   › **Touch:** take a hot or cool bath or shower, cuddle, soft blankets

   › **Taste:** eat or drink something cool, hot, crunchy, smooth, sweet

   › **Sound:** relaxing or upbeat music, talk to a friend, have TV on

   › **Smell:** scented candles, nature, cook, potpourri, aroma therapy

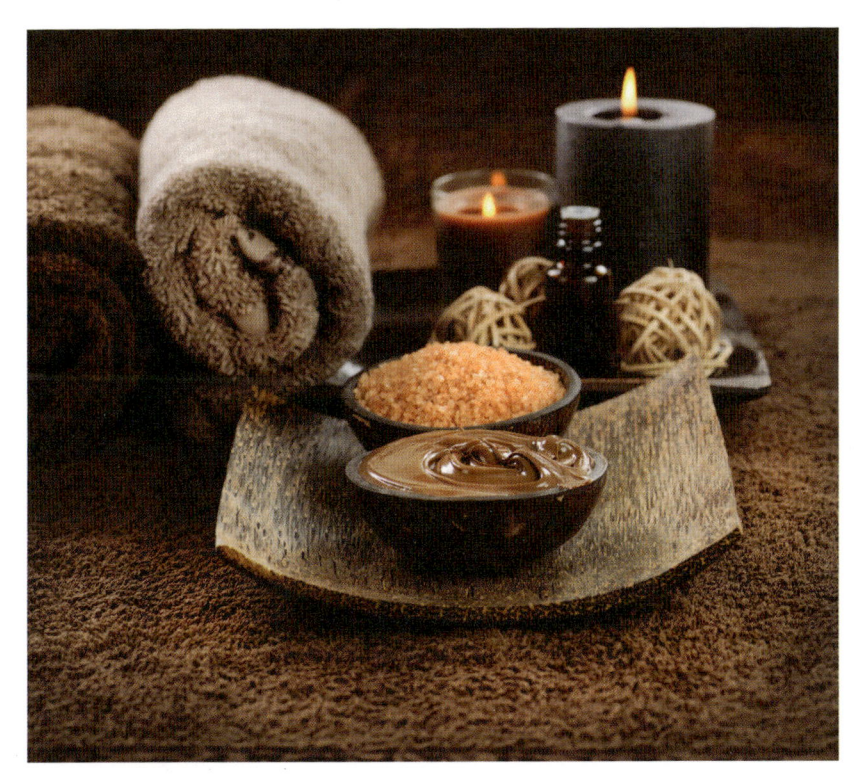

2. Utilize or visualize a safe place.

3. Visualize putting overwhelming thoughts, memories in a sealed container.

4. Do an activity that has you focus your mind; i.e., word search, puzzles.

5. Do a physical activity; i.e., sports, jogging, walking, exercise.

6. Express yourself verbally.

7. Write down your feelings in a journal.

8. Practice deep breathing exercises.

9. Listen to a relaxation tape/CD.

10. Get in touch with your personal spirituality.

11. Give yourself positive affirmations.

12. Remind yourself that you are in the present using a symbol of the present such as a stone, piece of jewelry, or any item you have received recently.

13. Become aware of your self-talk—change negative messages to positive ones.

14. Challenge your disturbing thoughts with the facts.

15. Find a grounding phrase (mantra), "I will get through this".

16. Deal with one issue at a time and break it into steps.

17. Keep it simple.

18. Say a prayer.

19. Make a phone call to someone.

20. Track your triggers.

21. Write down your problems; sort out what you can control and what you can't.

22. Go outside for some fresh air.

23. Talk to supportive people.

24. Practice some personal self-care such as massage, personal grooming.

25. Rock yourself in a rocking chair.

26. Do a progressive muscle relaxation.

Cognitive Behavioural Therapy (CBT)

At the Clairmont Digestive Clinic we believe in providing clients with practical tools to be able to problem-solve digestive needs independently. Our Digestive Health Therapist utilizes Cognitive Behavioural Therapy often referred to as (CBT) to support clients in navigating and exploring underlying issues or causes for Anxiety, Stress, or Tension within the body.

Cognitive Behaviour Therapy is a type of psychotherapy that looks at:

- How you think about yourself, the world, and other people
- How what you do affects your feelings and thoughts

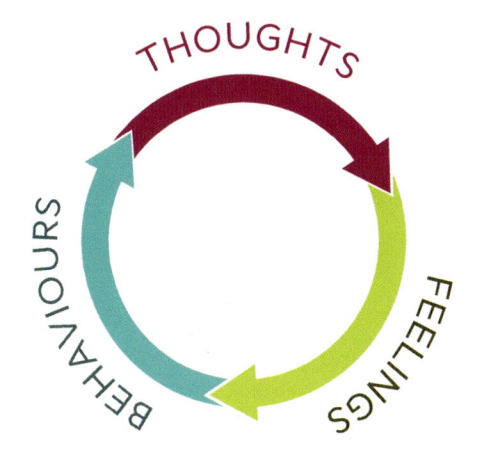

By making links between what we do, think, and feel, CBT can help us make changes in the way we think ("Cognitively") and the way we act, our ("Behaviours"). If we can identify the source of our problematic thoughts, and possible triggers we can begin exploring how incorporating coping strategies into your day-to-day life can support you approach your fears. If you are interested in beginning this process, book an appointment with our Digestive Health Therapist to further explore how your thoughts can be impacting your digestive health and overall well-being.

Adapted from: http://www.getselfhelp.co.uk/cbt.htm

My Personal Coping Plan

PERSONAL TRIGGERS

People:

Places:

Situations/Issues:

Time of day/year:

EARLY WARNING SIGNS

Physical Signs *(What changes do I notice in my body?)*:

Thoughts *(What am I saying to myself that is getting me more upset?)*:

COPING STRATEGIES —
WHEN I AM FEELING UPSET/STRESSED/ANXIOUS:

Helpful things for me to do are:

1.

2.

3.

4.

5.

6.

7.

8.

9.

10.

Things that are NOT helpful to do are:

People that are helpful are *(list name and number)*:

What I need from these people are:

1.

2.

3.

4.

5.

People that are NOT helpful are:

What I do NOT need from these people is:

Favourite Relaxation/Visualization Exercises are:

1.

2.

3.

4.

5.

Recommended Resources

The Complete Low-FODMAP Diet: A Revolutionary Plan for Managing IBS and Other Digestive Disorders by Sue Shepherd, PhD and Peter Gibson, MD

IBS: A Doctor's Plan for Chronic Digestive Troubles by Gerard Guillory, MD

10 Best Ever Anxiety Techniques Workbook by Margaret Wehrenberg

When the Body Says No by Gabor Mate

10 Mindful Minutes by Goldie Hawn

The Monash University App for Iphone Available at:
http://www.med.monash.edu/cecs/gastro/fodmap/

Chapter Two

The IBS MASTER PLAN Cookbook

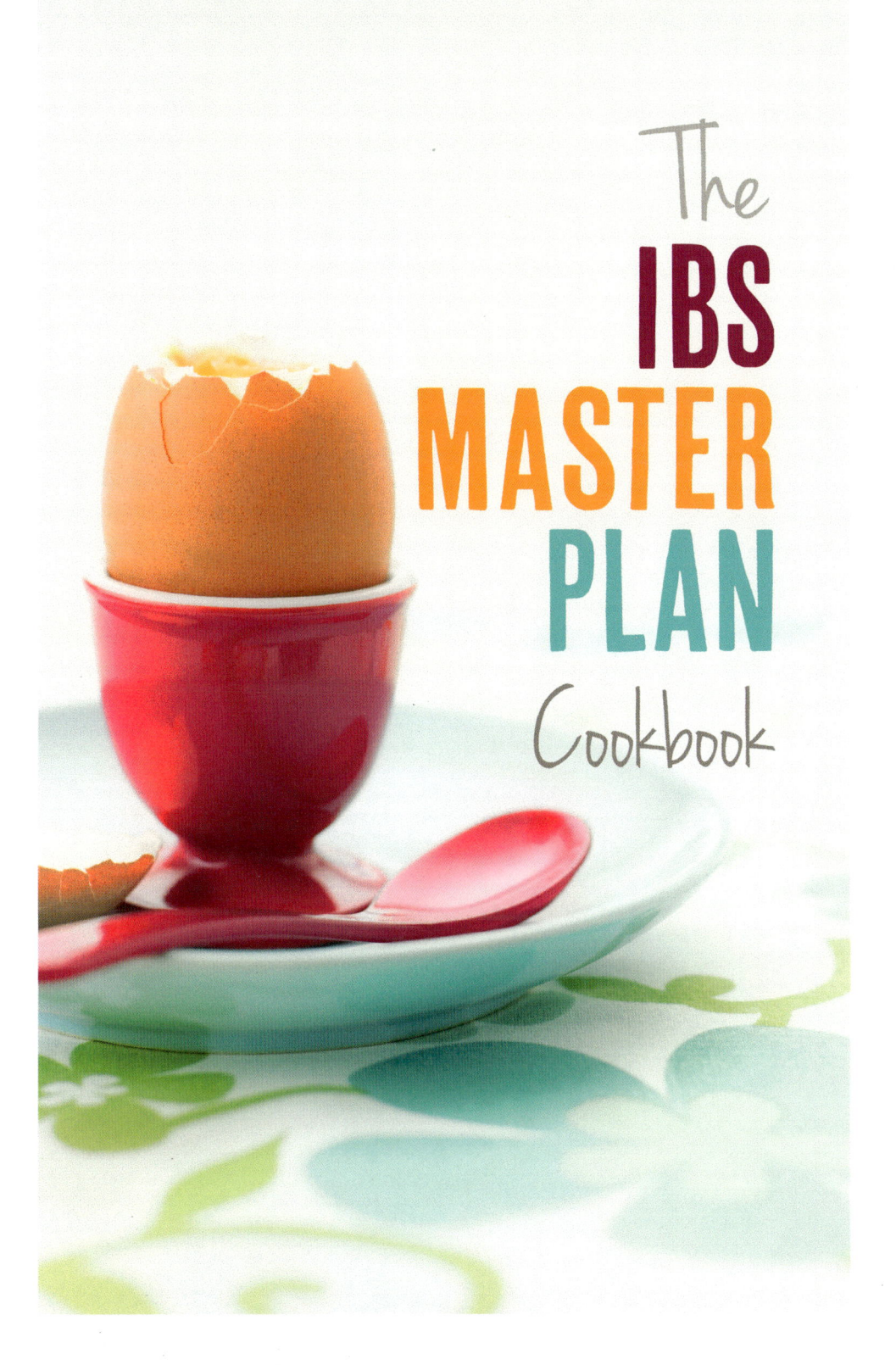

Breakfast

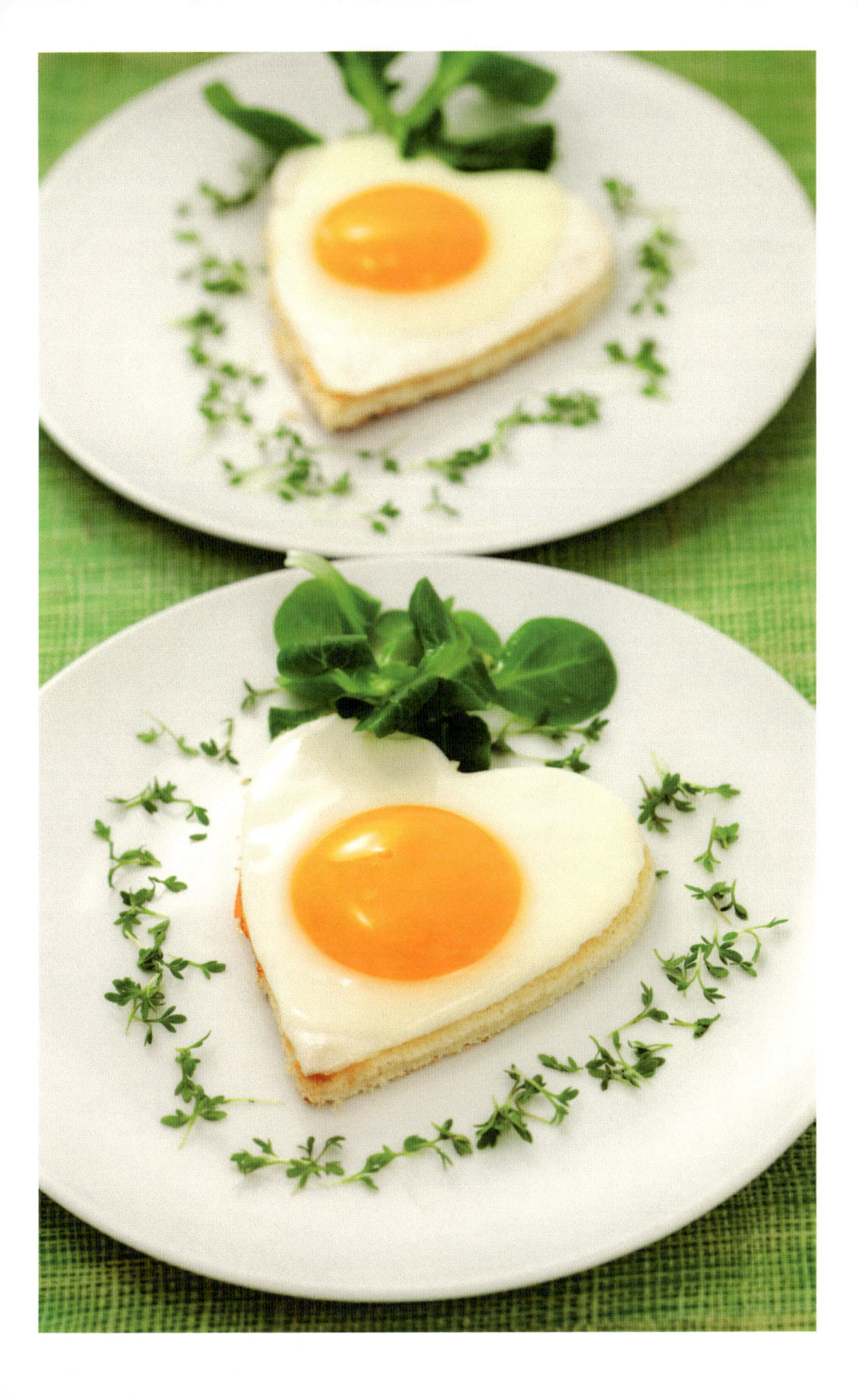

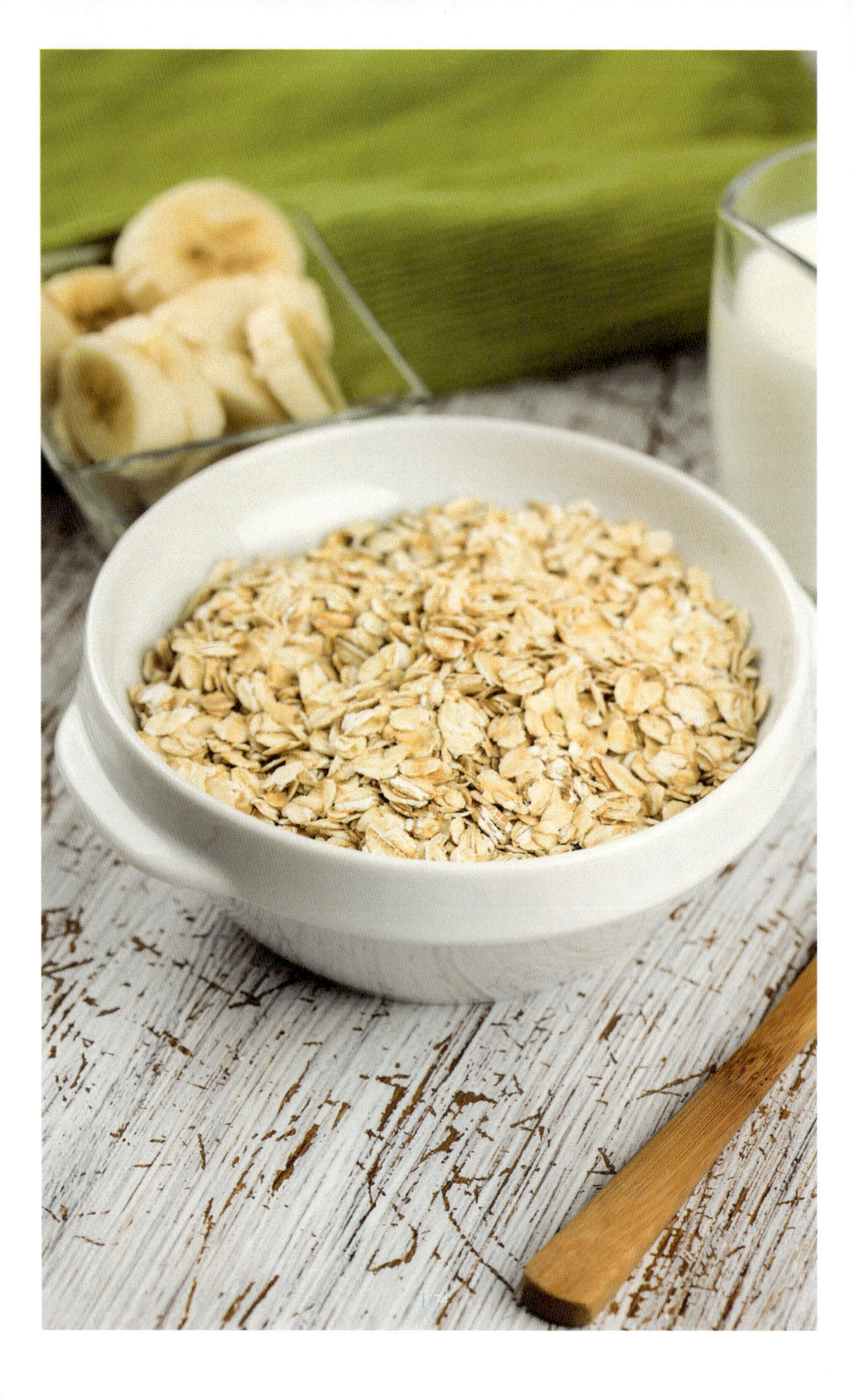

Amazing Oatmeal

Cook your oatmeal whatever way you please and add your ingredients for a perfectly balanced and filling morning meal.

These recipes make one serving

Strawberry Maple Oatmeal

INGREDIENTS

1 cup cooked oatmeal
(about ½ cup large flake oats dry)

½ cup strawberries

1 tbsp ground flax seeds

2 tbsp pumpkin seeds

1 tsp maple syrup

Blueberry Pecan Oatmeal

INGREDIENTS

1 cup cooked oatmeal
(about ½ cup large flake oats dry)

1 cup blueberries

1 tbsp ground flax seeds

2 tbsp pecans

1 tsp brown sugar

pinch of cinnamon

Banana Chocolate Oatmeal

INGREDIENTS

1 cup cooked oatmeal
(about ½ cup large flake oats dry)

½ to 1 banana, sliced
(depending on size)

2 tbsp walnuts

½ tbsp dark chocolate chips
(dairy free)

Pinch of sugar or maple syrup
for a little sweetness

Kiwi Coconut Oatmeal

INGREDIENTS

1 cup cooked oatmeal
(about ½ cup large flake oats dry)

2 kiwi, diced

2 tbsp sesame seeds

1 tsp dried coconut flakes

1 tsp brown sugar

Sensational Smoothies

Quick and easy breakfast solutions to your busy mornings.
Just add all the ingredients to blender.
Blend until smooth.

These recipes make one serving

Strawberry Banana Smoothie

INGREDIENTS

1 cup almond milk

1 tbsp ground flax seeds

3 tbsp hulled hemp seeds

½ frozen banana

¼ cup frozen kale

½ cup frozen strawberries

Peanut Butter Banana Blueberry Smoothie

INGREDIENTS

1 cup almond milk

1 tbsp ground flax seeds

2 tbsp peanut butter

½ frozen banana

¼ cup frozen spinach

1 cup blueberries

Creamy Cantaloupe Coconut Smoothie

INGREDIENTS

1 cup almond milk

3 tbsp hulled hemp seeds

¼ cup vanilla coconut yogurt

1 frozen banana

½ cup diced cantaloupe

Note from the Kitchen:

Frozen greens will puree more smoothly than fresh. When you get your kale home, wash, chop, and freeze. Frozen fruit opposed to fresh will provide a thickened texture and coolness to your smoothie.

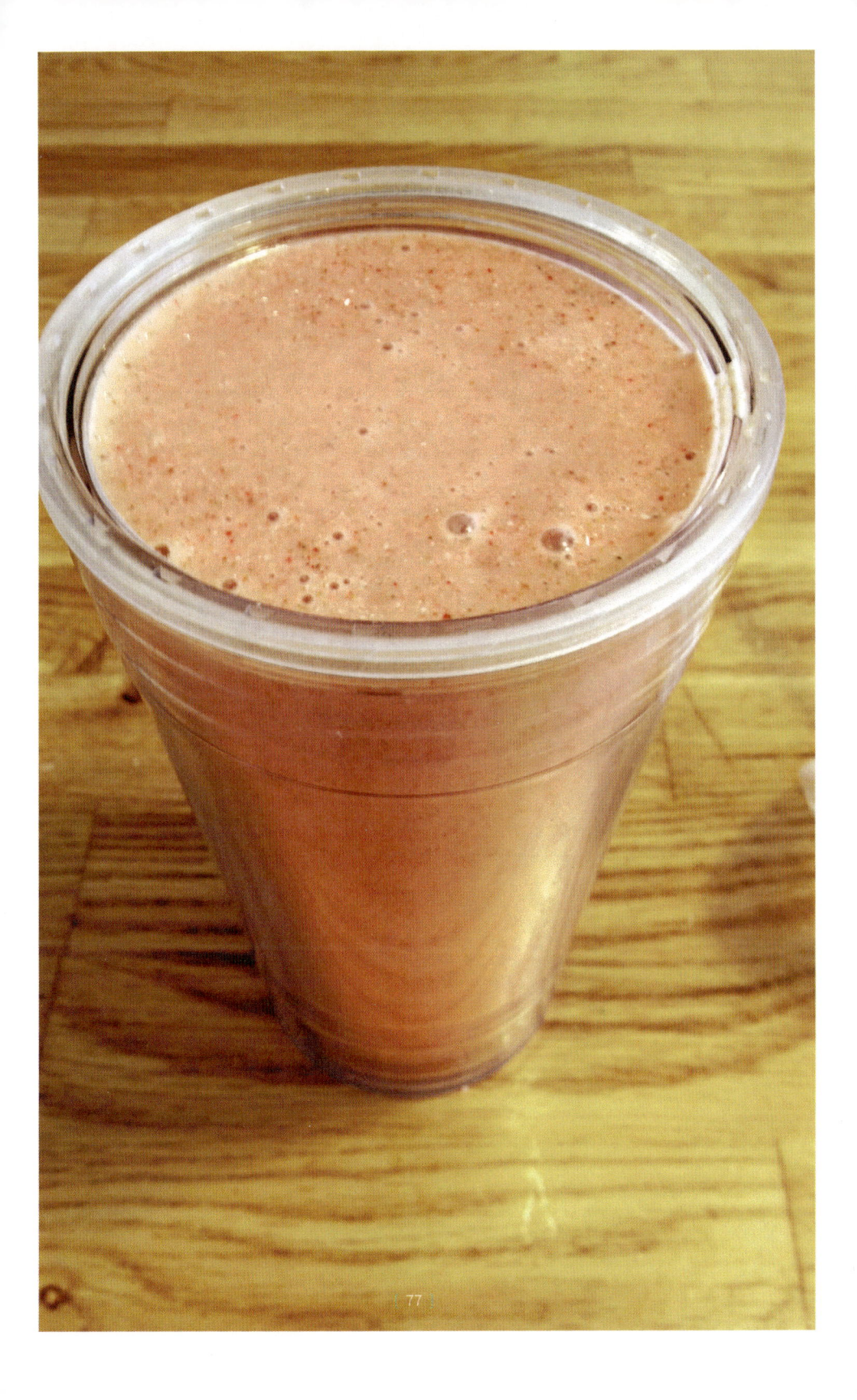

Tasty Toast Balanced Breakfast

Need your toast in the morning? Make sure to pair with protein and a little fibrous fruit to help you stay full all morning long!

High-Fibre Peanut Butter Breakfast

Toast 2 pieces high fibre gluten-free bread (like Udi's or Silver Hills bread) and serve with 2 tbsp peanut butter, 1 banana (sliced or served on the side), and one cup almond milk.

Eggs and Toast Breakfast

Toast 2 pieces gluten-free bread and serve with 1 whole egg + 1 egg white whatever way you like (poached/boiled/scrambled). Serve with sliced tomato and one cup almond milk.

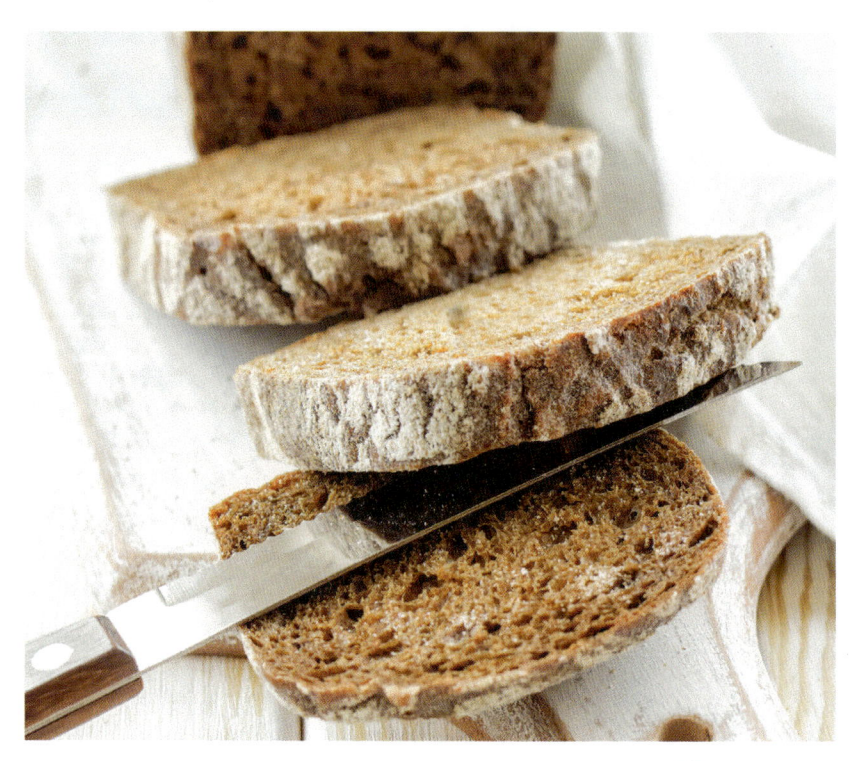

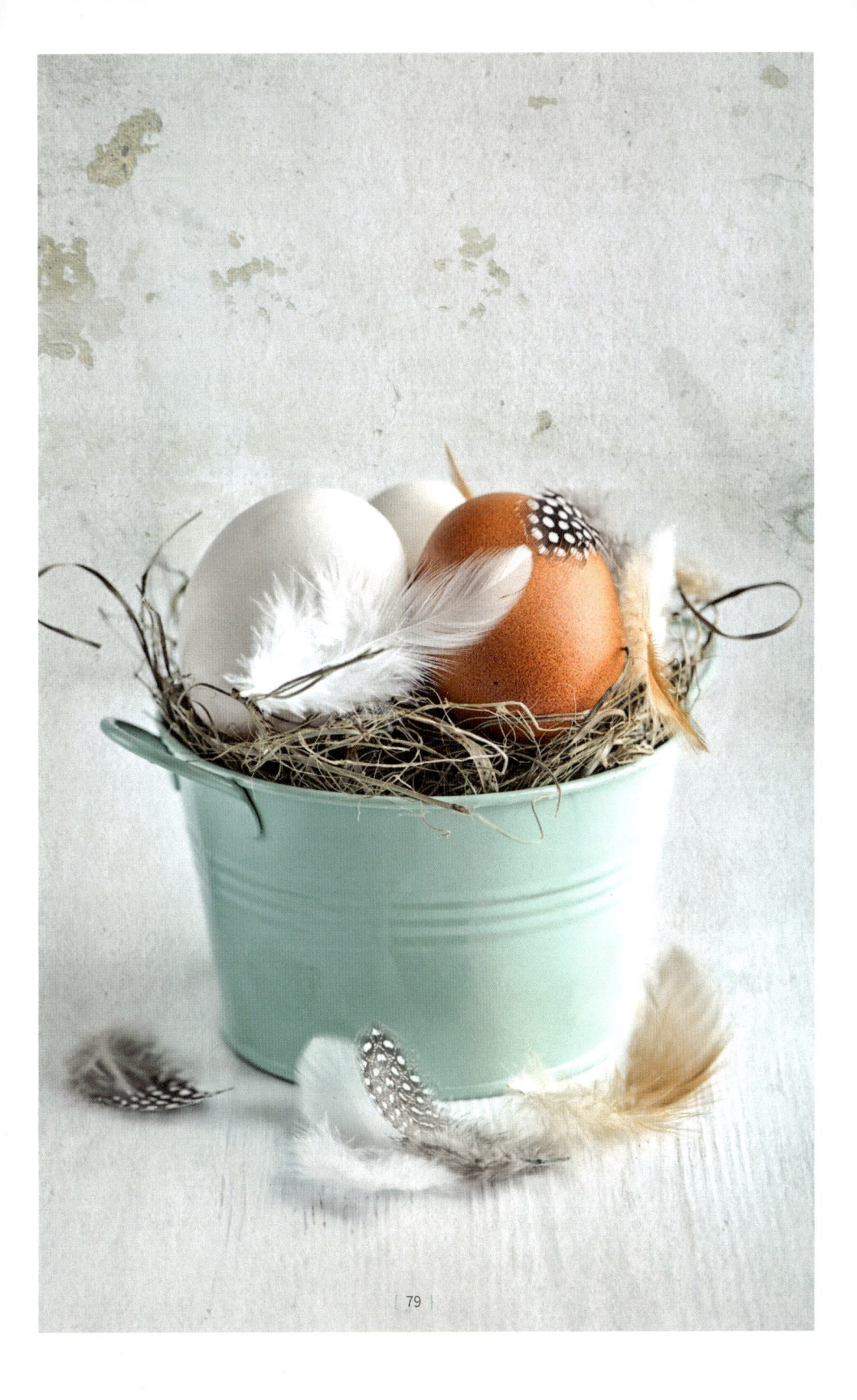

Fabulous French Toast and Pancakes

Cinnamon Pecan Banana French Toast

Makes 4 servings

Prep time: 2 minutes | Cook time: 5–6 minutes

INGREDIENTS

- 2 eggs
- 2 tsp cinnamon
- ¼ tsp vanilla extract
- 4 slices Udi's or other fresh, fluffy bread (do not use dense GF bread as it will not soak up eggs)
- Earth Balance margarine or non-GMO canola oil
- 4 tbsp pecans
- 1 banana, sliced
- 1 to 2 tsp maple syrup per serving

INSTRUCTIONS

1. Scramble the egg in a wide, flat bottomed bowl (think pasta plate) along with the cinnamon and vanilla.
2. Place the bread one slice at a time in the egg, flip to cover entire bread. Make sure each of the slices soak up all the egg so that none is leftover.
3. Warm a non-stick skillet over medium heat and add the margarine or oil. Place the egg soaked bread on the skillet and cook 2 to 3 minutes per side until slightly brown and toasty.
4. Serve on plate with pecans, bananas, and maple syrup.

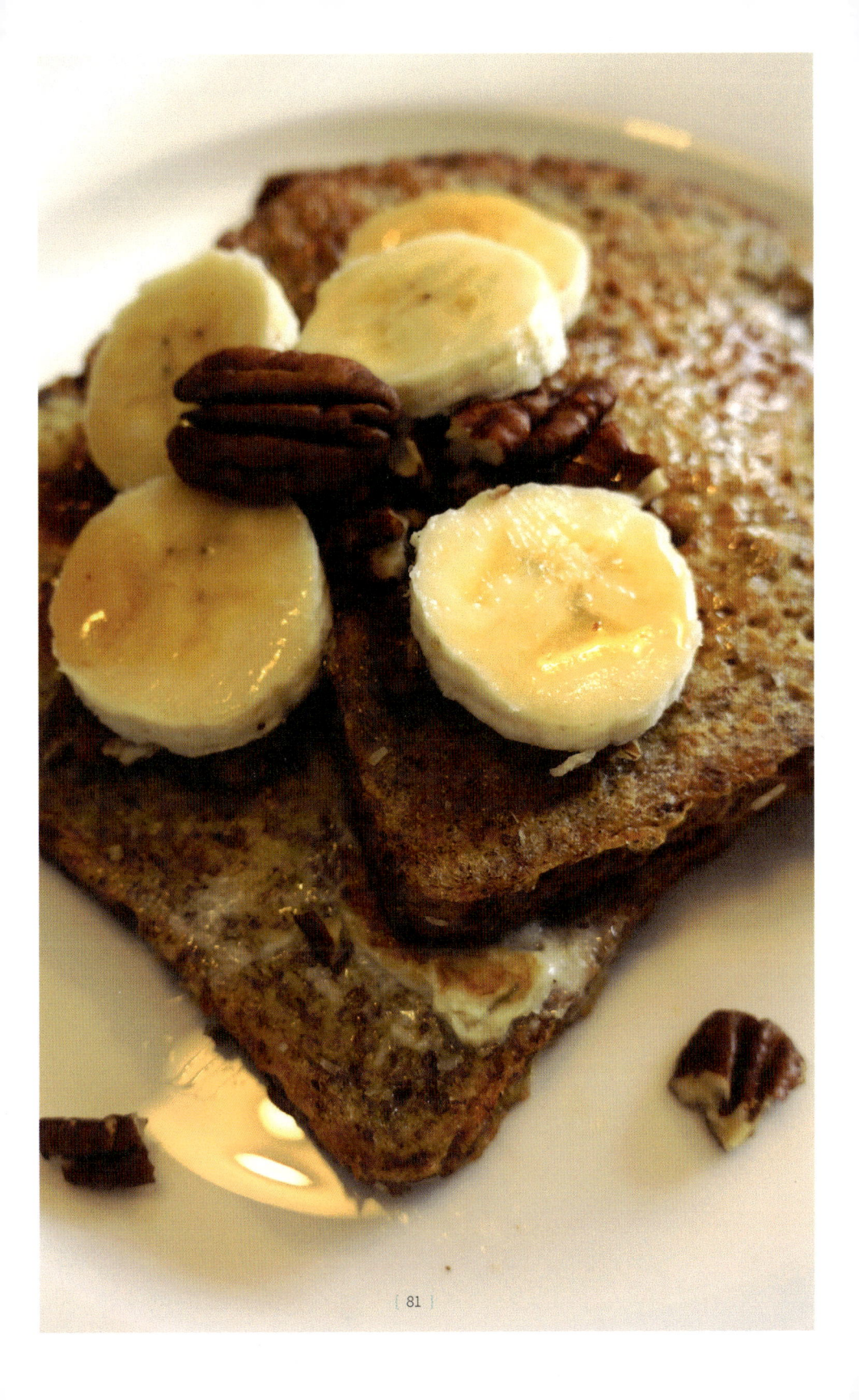

Raspberry Coconut French Toast

Makes 2 servings

Prep time: 2 minutes | Cook time: 5–6 minutes

INGREDIENTS

2 eggs

1 tsp cinnamon

¼ tsp coconut extract/flavouring

1 tsp brown sugar

4 slices Udi's or other fresh, fluffy bread (do not use dense GF bread as it will not soak up eggs)

Earth Balance margarine or non-GMO canola oil

1 ½ cup raspberries

3 tbsp hemp seeds

2 tsp dried coconut flakes

2 tsp brown sugar

INSTRUCTIONS

1. Scramble the egg in a wide, flat bottomed bowl (think pasta plate) along with the cinnamon, coconut flavouring, and ½ tsp brown sugar. Place the bread one slice at a time in the egg, flip to cover entire bread. Make sure each of the slices soak up all the egg so that none is leftover.

2. Warm a non-stick skillet over medium heat and add the margarine or oil. Place the egg soaked bread on the skillet and cook 2 to 3 minutes per side until slightly brown and toasty.

3. Serve on plate with raspberries, hemp seeds, coconut flakes, and brown sugar.

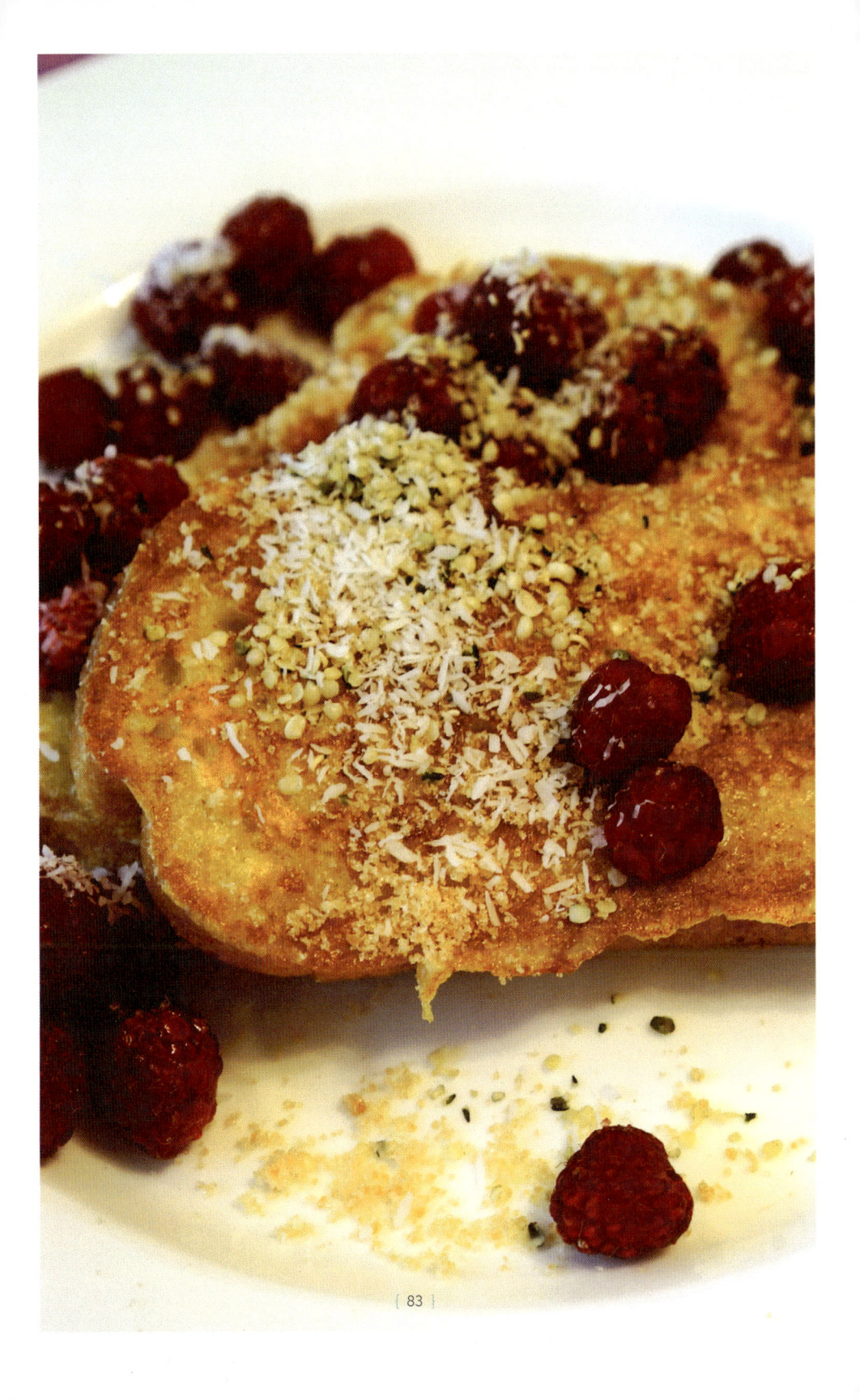

Wild Blueberry Pancakes

Makes 4 servings

Prep time: 5 minutes | Cook time: 5–10 minutes

INGREDIENTS

- ¾ cup rice flour
- ¼ cup almond flour/meal
- ¼ cup ground flax
- 2 tsp cinnamon
- 1 ½ tsp baking soda
- Pinch of salt
- ½ cup almond milk
- 1 tsp coconut oil
- 1 egg
- 4 cups blueberries

INSTRUCTIONS

1. In a large bowl, mix together the dry ingredients.
2. In a separate bowl, mix together the wet ingredients, leaving out the blueberries. Add the wet ingredients to the dry ingredients. Stir until just combined.
3. Warm a large non-stick skillet on medium-low heat. Add 1 tsp canola, olive, or coconut oil, or vegan margarine to the pan. Scoop about ⅛ to ¼ cup of the batter out and drop on the pan. Sprinkle a couple of blueberries into the pancake. Cook pancakes 2 to 3 minutes per side until golden brown and cooked through. Serve with the remainder of the blueberries.

Note from the Kitchen:

If making a large batch of pancakes, keep those that are cooked already warm in the oven at 225°F until all are ready to serve.

Pumpkin Oat Pancakes

Makes 4 servings

Prep time: 5 minutes | Cook time: 5–10 minutes

INGREDIENTS

- ½ cup rice flour
- ½ cup large flake oats
- ¼ cup sweet white sorghum flour
- ¼ cup potato starch
- ⅛ cup chickpea flour
- 2 tbsp cup ground flax
- 2 tbsp brown sugar
- 1 tbsp baking powder
- 1 tsp cinnamon
- ½ tsp nutmeg
- ⅛ tsp cloves
- Pinch of salt
- 1 cup almond milk
- 2 tbsp canola, olive, or coconut oil
- 1 egg
- ½ cup pureed pumpkin
- 1–2 tsp maple syrup per person

INSTRUCTIONS

1. In a large bowl, mix together the dry ingredients.
2. In a separate bowl, mix together the wet ingredients. Add the wet ingredients to the dry ingredients. Stir until just combined.
3. Warm a large non-stick skillet on medium-low heat. Add 1 tsp canola, olive, or coconut oil to the pan or vegan margarine. Scoop about ⅛ to ¼ cup of the batter out and drop on the pan. Cook pancakes 2 to 3 minutes per side until golden brown and cooked through. Serve with maple syrup as desired.

Note from the Kitchen:

If making a large batch of pancakes, keep those that are cooked already warm in the oven at 225°F until all are ready to serve.

Soups, Salads, and Sides

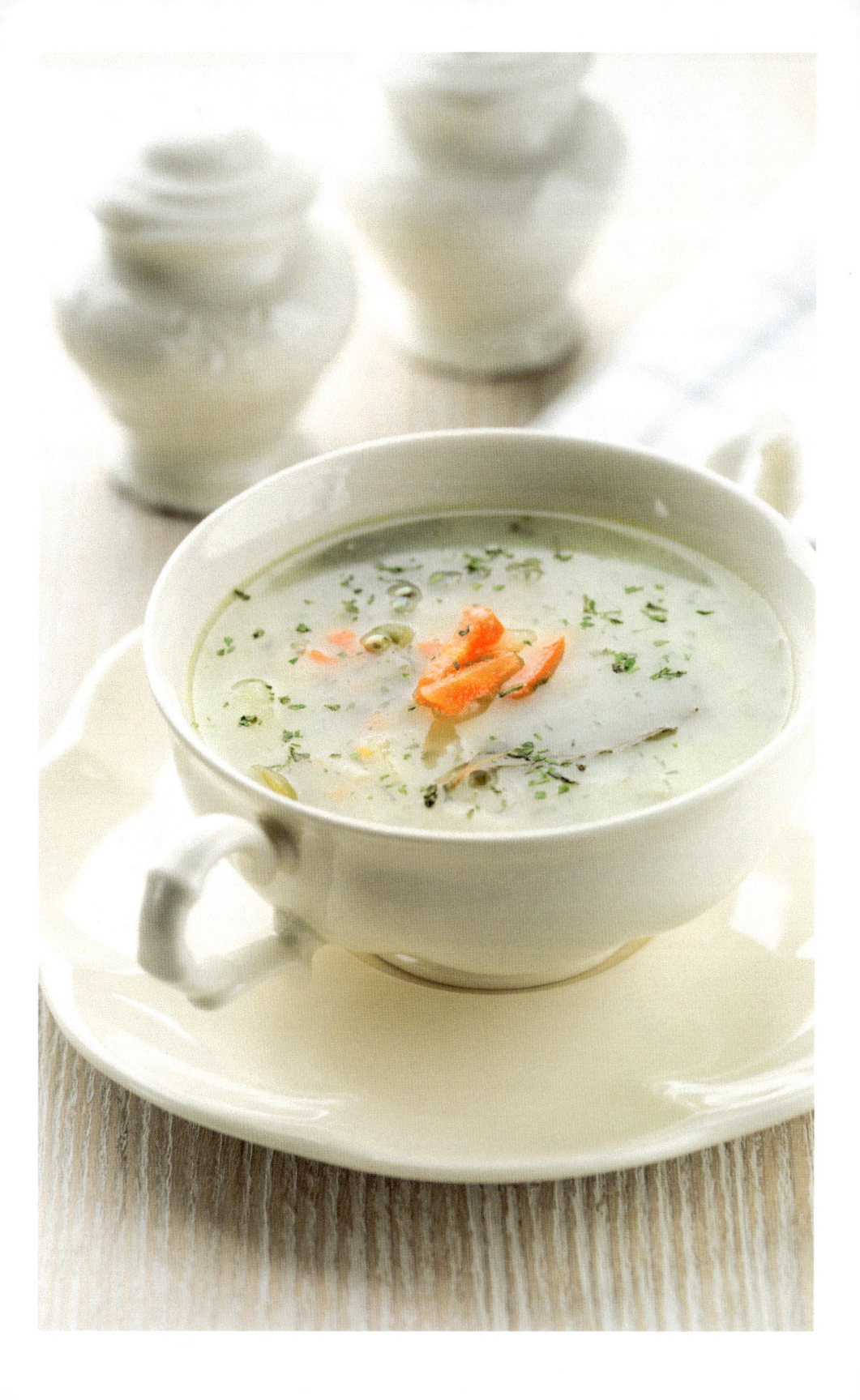

Stupendous Superfood Minestrone

Makes 4 servings

Prep time: 15 minutes | Cook time: 30–40 minutes

INGREDIENTS

2 strips bacon or pancetta

2 tsp olive oil

2 sticks celery, diced small

1 carrot, diced small

½ cup fennel, diced small

2 cups potato, diced small

4 cups water

2 large (about 2 cups) tomatoes, diced large

¼ tsp EACH sage, parsley, and oregano

*¼ tsp chili flakes *optional*

¼ cup quinoa (uncooked)

2 cups kale, shredded

1 cup canned chickpeas, drained, rinsed

Salt & pepper

Olive oil

Lemon

*Parmesan Reggiano cheese, grated *optional*

INSTRUCTIONS

1. Place a large metal pot on medium heat. Add diced bacon or pancetta and cook until half way done, about 4 to 5 minutes. Add olive oil—use less if some of the fat released from the bacon is kept in the pot. Add the celery, carrot, and fennel. Cook for 3 to 5 minutes until vegetables start to caramelize (turns slightly brown). Add water, potato, tomato, sage, parsley, oregano, quinoa, and chili flakes if using. Bring to a boil, cover and simmer for 15 minutes.

2. Add kale and chickpeas and cook for 5 minutes more. Season with salt and pepper to taste. Serve with a little drizzle of olive oil, squeeze of fresh lemon, and a little cheese if desired.

Note from the Kitchen:

Instead of quinoa you can use rice or pasta. You can also add or replace the chickpeas with other proteins like leftover chicken, sausage (don't use the bacon), or crumbled tempeh.

Note about Digestion:

Celery over ½ stick in serving size is moderate in the FODMAP polyols, so be sure to stick to the serving in this recipe if this is a trigger for you. Although garlic is high in the FODMAP fructans, you can simmer a few cloves in the oil at the beginning of the recipe, just be sure to remove them before you add other ingredients. Alternatively, you can use garlic-infused olive oil. For some, stock can cause symptoms—if you can tolerate in small amounts cut the water in half and replace with a good quality store bought or homemade stock. *Epicure Selections* makes a good powdered variety.

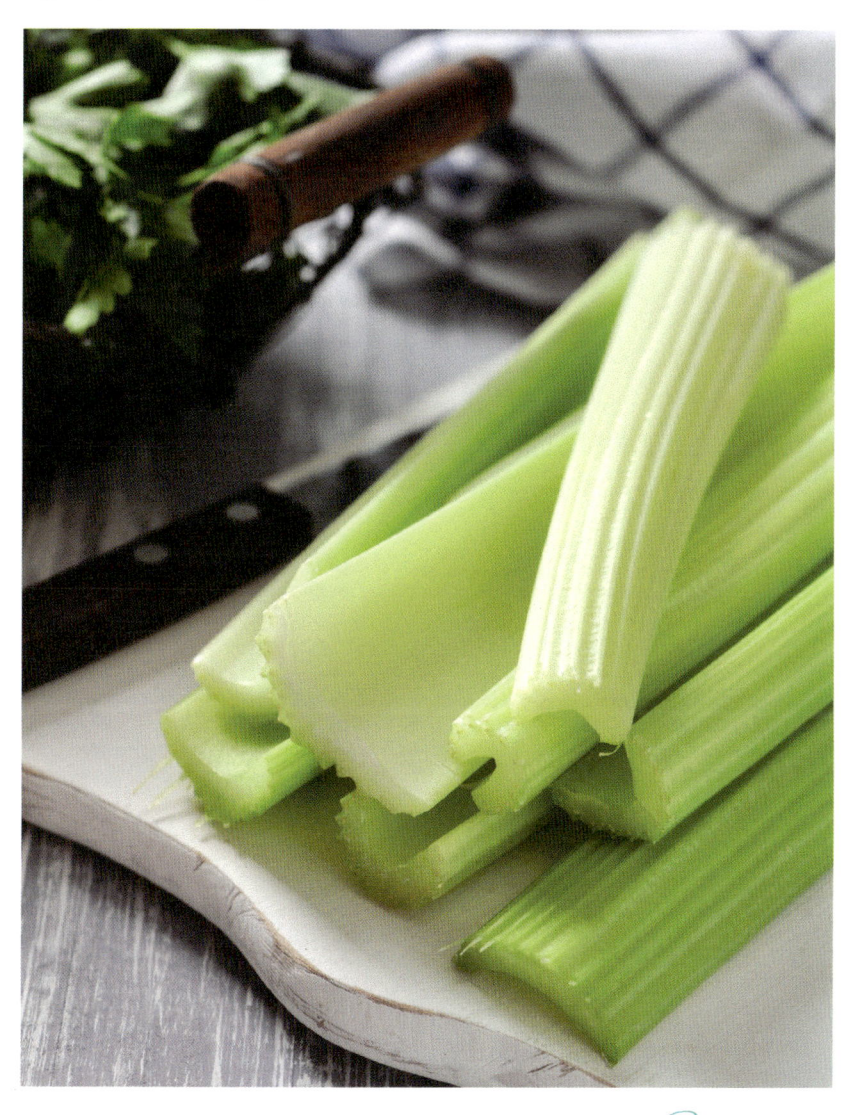

Hearty Wholesome Harvest Soup

Makes 4 servings

Prep time: 15 minutes | Cook time: 30–40 minutes

INGREDIENTS

2 tsp olive oil

2 sticks celery, diced medium

1 carrot, diced medium

½ cup fennel bulb, diced medium

2 parsnips, diced medium

3 small (about 1 cup) potatoes, halved, then quartered

½ small (about 1 cup) butternut squash

3 cups water

3 cups vegetable or chicken stock

½ tsp EACH sage and rosemary

1 bay leaf

¼ tsp cinnamon (more if you like)

Pinch of salt and pepper (more to taste)

1 block (about 250 g) tempeh, preferably organic

1 cup canned lentils, drained, rinsed

2 cups spinach, diced

INSTRUCTIONS

1. Place a large metal pot on medium heat. Add olive oil, celery, carrot, fennel, parsnips, potatoes, squash, water, stock, herbs, cinnamon, salt, and pepper to pot. Bring to a boil, cover, and simmer for 15 minutes.

2. Meanwhile, in a small pot of boiling water add the tempeh. Simmer on a low boil for 10 minutes (to remove some of the fermented flavour). Remove from pot, cut into 12 smaller blocks, and allow to cook for 5 minutes. Once cool, crumble into small pieces.

3. When soup has cooked for 15 minutes, the tempeh should be ready. Add the crumbled tempeh and lentils to the soup. Cook for 10 to 15 minutes more until vegetables are tender.

4. Season with salt and pepper to taste. Add spinach immediately before serving.

Note from the Kitchen:

Instead of tempeh, you could add ½ lb ground chicken or turkey to this soup.

Note about Digestion:

Celery over ½ stick in serving size is moderate in the FODMAP polyols and butternut squash >¼ cup serving is moderate in fructans. Be sure to be mindful of these ingredients and reduce or eliminate if they are symptom triggers. Although garlic is high in the FODMAP fructans, you can simmer a few cloves in the oil at the beginning of the recipe, just be sure to remove them before you add other ingredients. Alternatively, you can use garlic-infused olive oil. For some, stock can cause symptoms—if you can tolerate in small amounts cut the water in half and replace with a good quality store bought or homemade stock. *Epicure Selections* makes a good powdered variety.

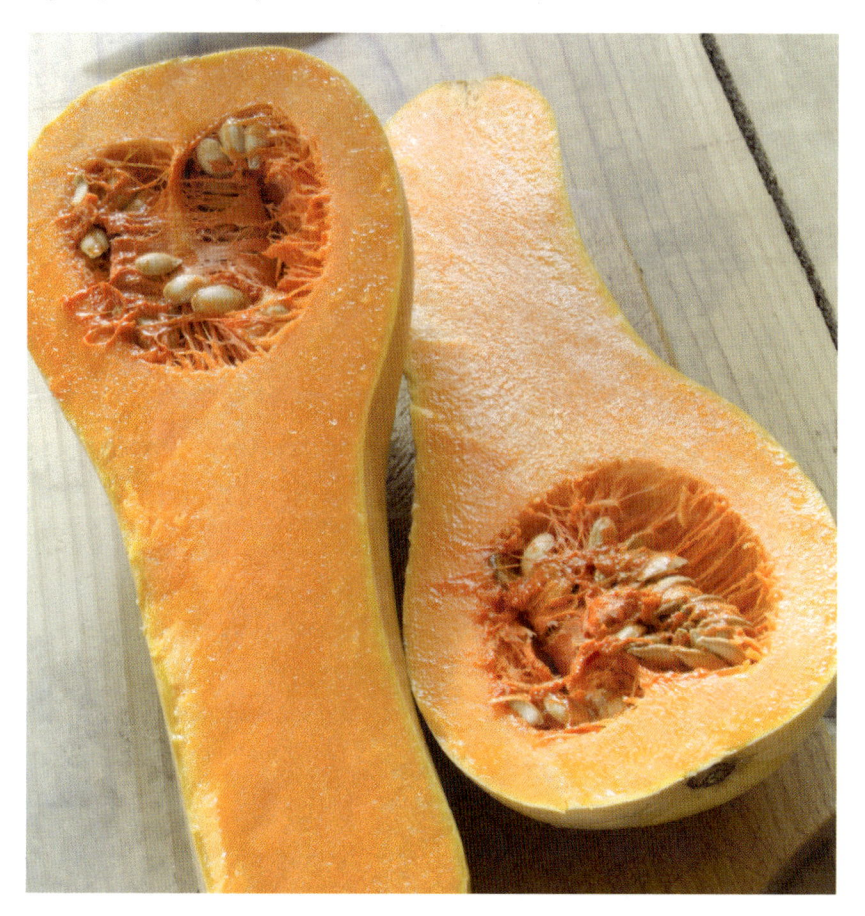

Roasted Red Pepper Pasta Salad

Makes 4 servings

Prep time: 20 minutes | Cook time: 25 minutes

INGREDIENTS

3 cups penne pasta (gluten free), uncooked

2 large red bell peppers, cored, seeded, and quartered

1 medium yellow zucchini, cut into 1 cm thick slices

1 small fennel bulb, halved

1 ½ tbsp olive oil

Salt and pepper to taste

4 cups kale, chopped

1 cup canned chickpeas, rinsed and drained

6 tbsp pine nuts

2 cups cherry tomatoes

Juice of 1 lemon

1 tbsp white wine vinegar

1 tsp dried thyme

1 tsp dried parsley

Big handful of fresh basil leaves, chopped

Pinch of cayenne and/or red pepper flakes *optional

Feta or parmesan cheese, to serve

INSTRUCTIONS

1. Preheat the oven to 425°F.
2. Place a large pot of water on the stove, cover, and bring to a boil. Meanwhile, toss the peppers, zucchini, and fennel in 1 tablespoon of the olive oil and season with salt and pepper. Place onto a lined baking sheet and roast in the oven, flipping once during cooking, until somewhat tender, about 20 to 25 minutes. Set aside to cool before dicing the vegetables into ½-inch size pieces and transferring to a large bowl.
3. Meanwhile, cook the pasta according to package directions, adding the kale during the last minute of cooking. When pasta is al dente, drain it with the kale and toss with the remaining olive oil. Spread on a large platter or baking sheet to cool.
4. Add cooled pasta to the cooled vegetables and add the rest of the ingredients, tossing gently. Serve sprinkled with a little cheese as desired.

Note from the Kitchen:

This pasta salad also tastes lovely with diced chicken breast, sausage, or shrimp. You can substitute one of these alternative proteins with the chickpeas or include both in the meal. You can also substitute any kind of nut or seed you like for the pine nuts.

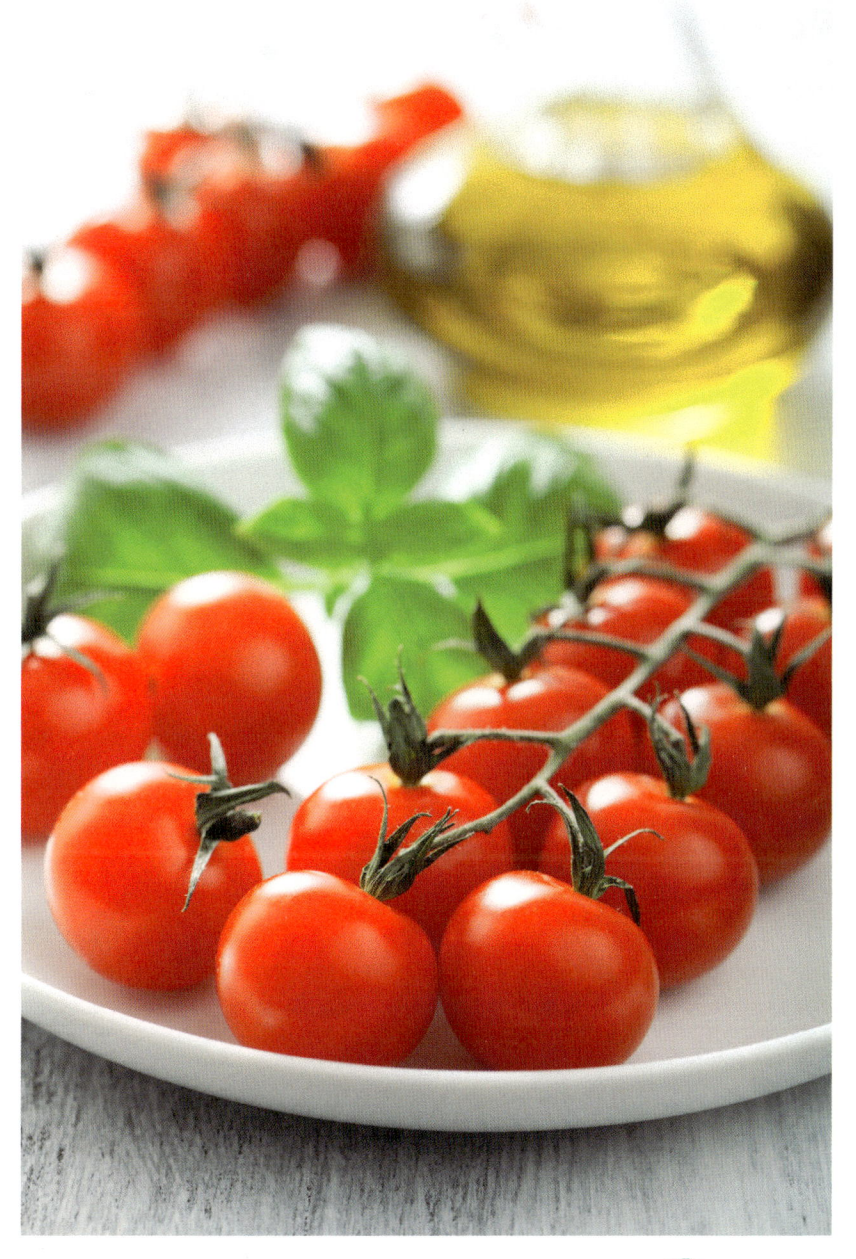

Lemon Dill Tuna Pasta Salad

Makes 4 servings

Prep time: 10 minutes | Cook time: 15 minutes

INGREDIENTS

2 cups uncooked pasta (penne or shells) (gluten free)

4 large eggs

1 can tuna, in water, drained

2 cups finely shredded kale or spinach

¼ cup fennel, minced

4 cups cherry tomatoes, halved

1 large (about 2 cups) cucumber, seeded and diced

1 tbsp olive oil

2 tbsp mayonnaise

1 tsp Dijon mustard

Pinch of cayenne

1 tsp dill, dried OR 1 tbsp fresh

Juice of ½ to 1 lemon as desired

Salt and pepper to taste

INSTRUCTIONS

1. Bring a large pot of water to a boil. Add gluten-free pasta, preferably *Tinkyada* or *Le Venezianne* brand, to the water and simmer according to package directions and desired texture is reached.

2. Meanwhile, boil eggs in a smaller pot—hard boiled is 10 minutes.

3. Place kale, fennel, tomatoes, and cucumbers in a large bowl. Add tuna and mix together. Peel and chop eggs and add to bowl. Toss cooked pasta in olive oil and add to bowl. Add mayonnaise, Dijon, cayenne, dill, and lemon. Season with salt and pepper to taste. Serve warm or cold.

Note from the Kitchen:

You can also use fresh tuna or salmon in this recipe. Just grill or bake until cooked through. Allow to cool and flake with a fork. Use about 250 to 300 grams uncooked fish.

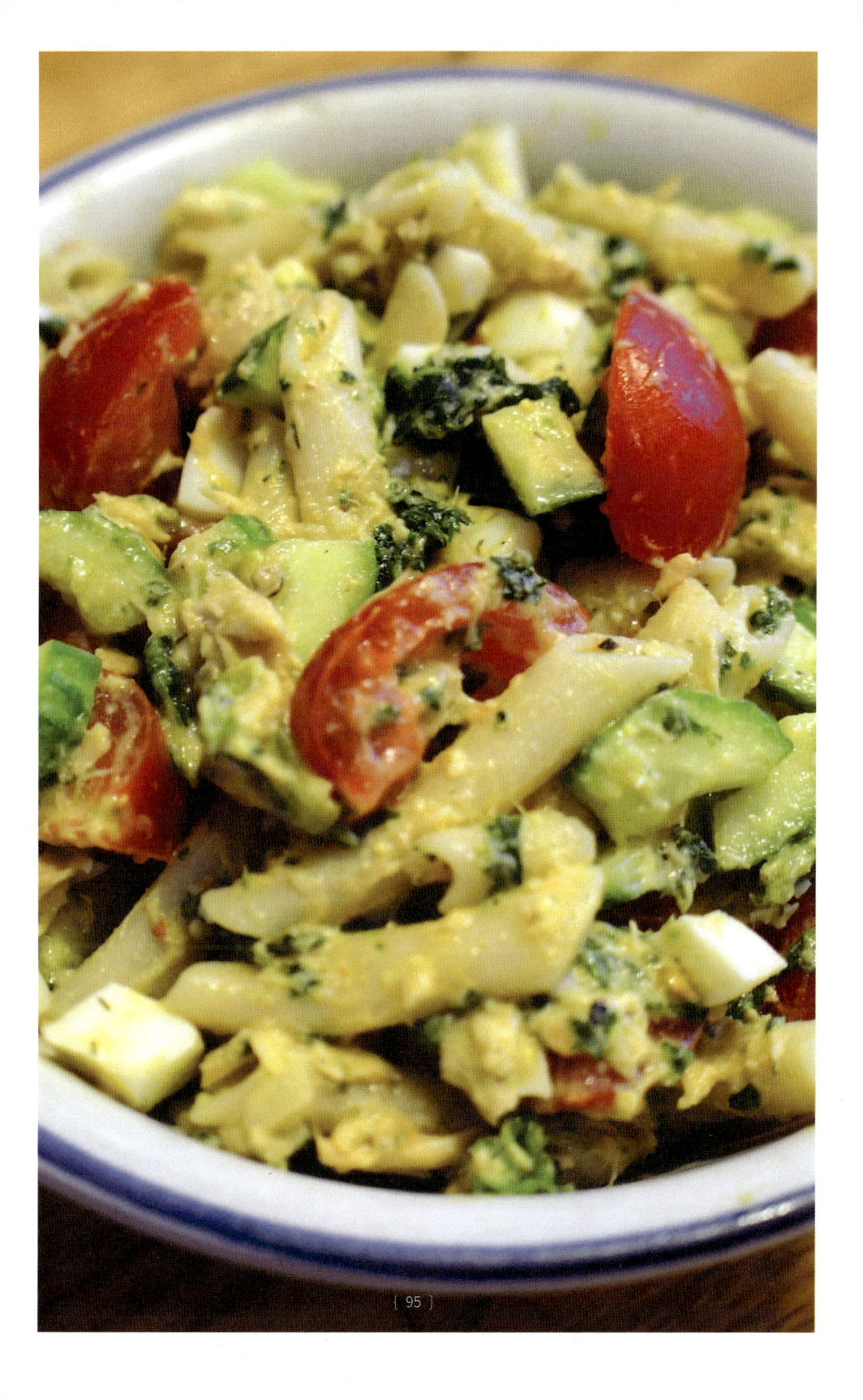

Roasted Vegetable Lentil Salad

Makes 4 servings

Prep time: 10 minutes | Cook time: 20 minutes

INGREDIENTS

2 cups quinoa, uncooked

3 cups water

1 medium green zucchini, diced (about 2 cups)

2 large yellow peppers (about 2 cups), diced

1 ½ tbsp olive oil

1 tsp dried basil

1 tsp dried parsley

2 cups cherry tomatoes, halved

1 ½ cups canned lentils, drained and rinsed

½ cup walnut pieces

1 ½ tbsp balsamic vinegar

Salt and pepper to taste

INSTRUCTIONS

1. Preheat the oven to 425°F.

2. In a medium saucepan, combine the quinoa and water. Cover, bring to a boil, reduce heat, and simmer 15 minutes until tender. Remove the lid and fluff with a fork. Set aside.

3. Meanwhile, combine the zucchini and pepper in a bowl and toss with the olive oil. Place on a lined baking sheet and roast for 10 minutes. Remove vegetables from the oven. Stir in the basil, parsley, and tomatoes and return to the oven to cook for another 5 to 10 minutes, or until all vegetables are cooked through and tender.

4. Combine the quinoa, roasted vegetables (be sure to add all liquid from the roasting pan), lentils, walnuts, balsamic vinegar, salt, and pepper to taste. Toss well and serve.

Note from the Kitchen:

Adapt this salad to include other "easy to digest" vegetables like eggplant, fennel, green beans, and carrots. Adjust your cooking time depending on the vegetables you roast. Try fresh herbs for a different flavour—add right before serving.

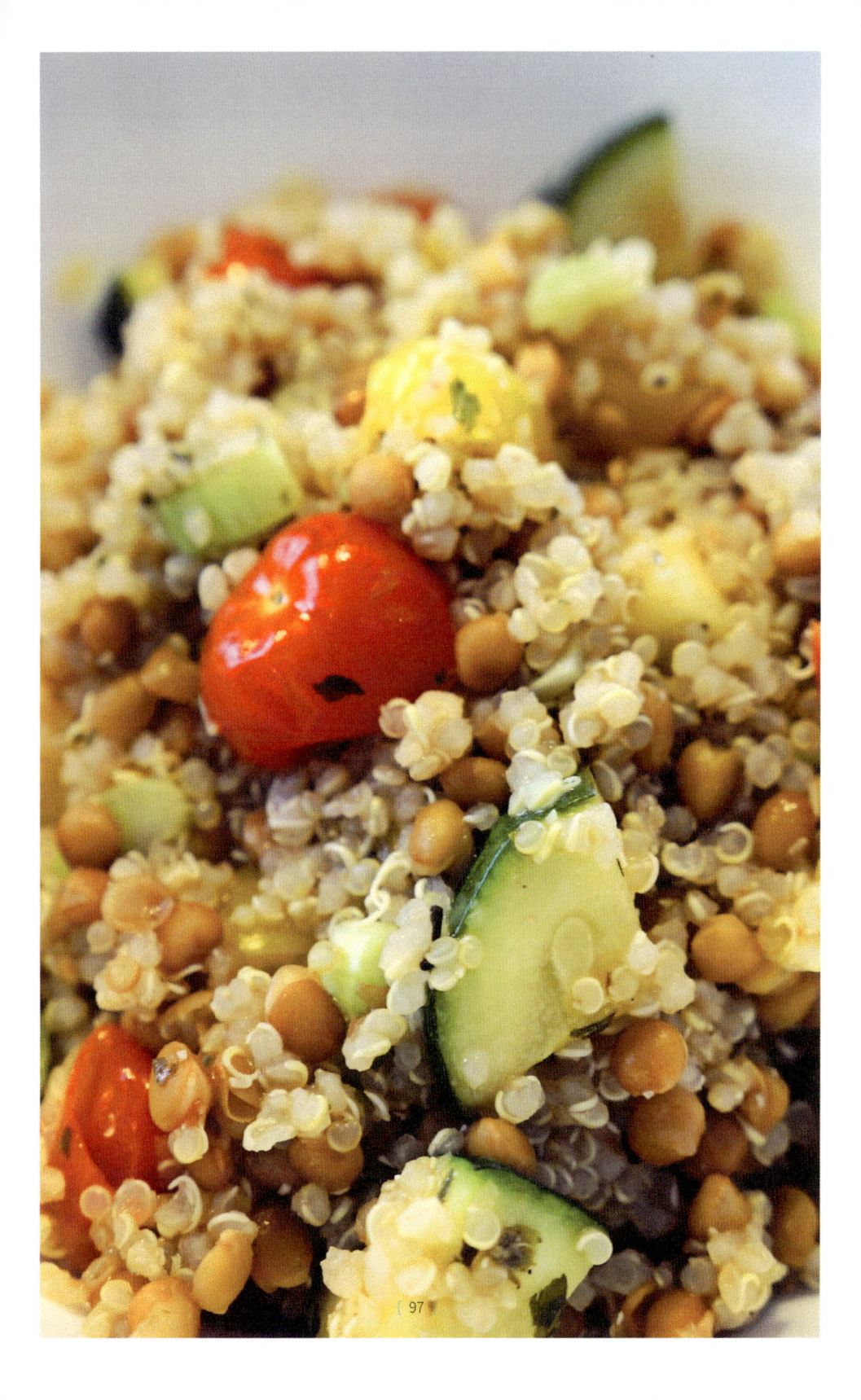

Leafy Italian Salad with Quinoa

Makes 4 servings

Prep time: 10 minutes | Cook time: 15 minutes

INGREDIENTS

1 cup quinoa, uncooked

1 ½ cups water or low-sodium vegetable or chicken stock

4 cups baby spinach or mixed greens

Handful of sprouts or micro-greens

2 cups cherry tomatoes, halved

2 roasted red peppers, sliced

1 cup canned chickpeas, drained and rinsed

½ cup pine nuts

Drizzle of olive oil

Light drizzle of balsamic vinegar

Fresh squeeze of lemon

Salt and pepper to taste

*Handful of fresh basil *optional*

INSTRUCTIONS

1. In a small pot combine the quinoa and water. Bring to a boil. Cover, reduce heat, and simmer with lid on for 15 minutes. Consider adding 1 tsp of the *Epicure* chicken stock to quinoa, which adds just a little flavour, without adding too much salt.

2. Meanwhile, toss together the spinach, sprouts, tomatoes, peppers, chickpeas, and pine nuts and divide into 4 serving bowls. Top each with the cooked quinoa. Drizzle olive oil, balsamic vinegar, and lemon onto each salad and season to taste with salt and pepper. Finish with the basil as desired.

Note from the Kitchen:

This is a great recipe for leftover quinoa. You can also use other low FODMAP vegetables, or nuts and seeds, like pecans, walnuts, peanuts, or sunflower seeds as desired.

Note about Digestion:

Chickpeas are high in the FODMAP oligos. If this is a trigger food for you, ensure you follow the recipe and consume no more than ¼ cup in a meal. Even in this small amount, they may be bothersome. You can substitute lentils, nuts/seeds, eggs, chicken, fish, or any other protein.

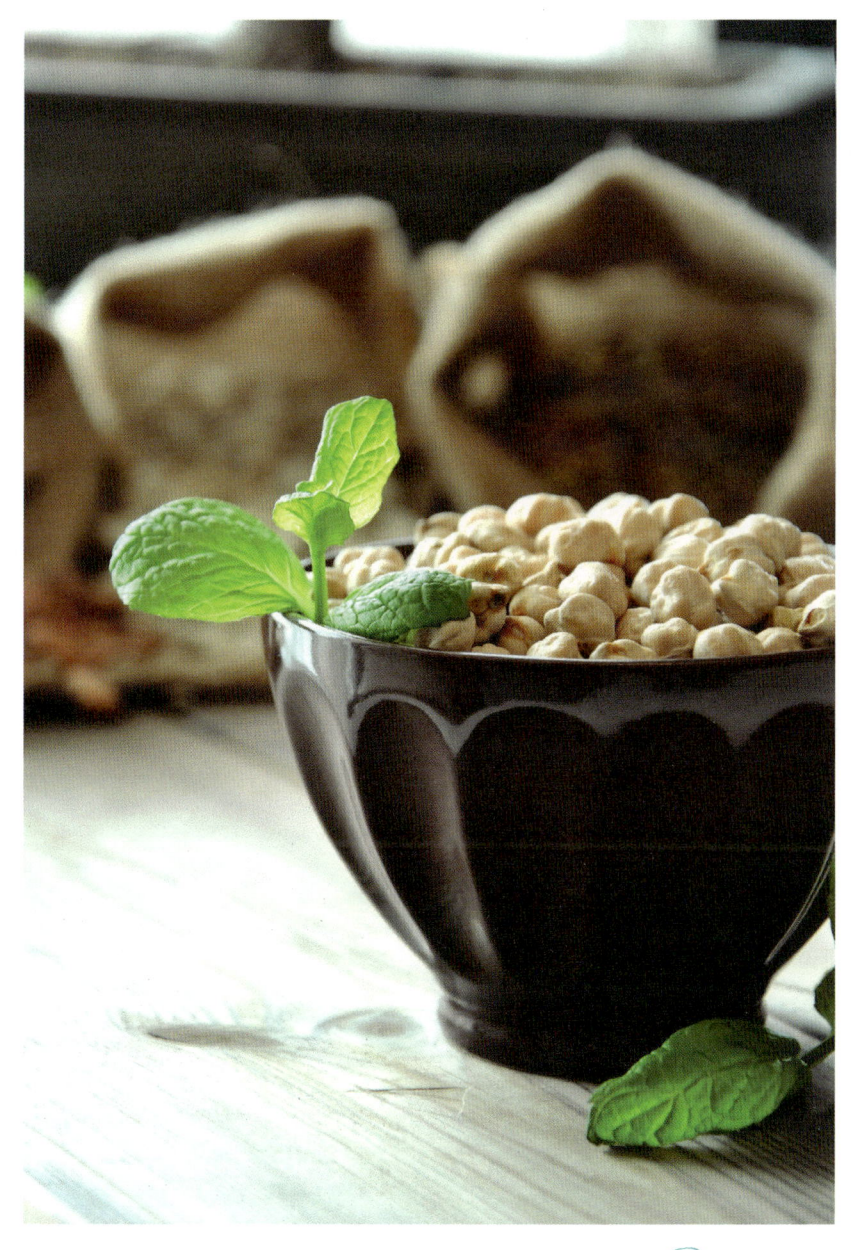

Simple Rice Paper Salad Rolls

Makes 4 servings (about 2 to 3 rolls per person)

Prep time: 20 minutes | Cook time: 5 minutes

INGREDIENTS

½ pack (½ lb) vermicelli or other rice noodle

Sesame oil

Rice paper sheets

Any of the following protein sources:

Chicken breast (cooked and diced)

Shrimp (cooked and whole)

Marinated and grilled tofu (cut into long strips)

Ground pork, beef, or chicken (cooked)

Salmon or tuna (canned or cooked), flaked

Any of the following vegetables:

Shredded lettuce or other greens

Micro-greens like alfalfa sprouts

Thinly sliced bell peppers

Thinly sliced cucumbers

Grated carrots

Grated radishes

Fresh cilantro

Fresh lime

Homemade sweet chili sauce:

¼ cup rice or white vinegar

¼ cup water

2 tbsp white sugar

¼ tsp salt

1 tsp red chili paste, red chili flakes, OR hot pepper like jalapeno or serrano, diced very small

1 tsp corn starch

2 tbsp cold water

INSTRUCTIONS

1. Bring a large pot of water to a boil. Cook rice noodles for 2 to 5 minutes, or according to package directions. Drain and toss with a little sesame oil and set aside. Prepare and arrange all other ingredients so they are accessible for rolling.

2. Make the sauce by combing the vinegar and water in a small pot. Bring to a boil. Add the sugar, salt, chili paste or other hot pepper, and simmer for 3 to 5 minutes, until mixture starts to thicken. Whisk corn starch with 2 tbsp of cold water seperately until dissolved, then stir into the pot. Turn off heat and stir for 1 minute more. Transfer to a small bowl and allow to cool. Refrigerate until needed.

3. To make the rolls, dip the rice paper into a deep dish of warm water until soft, about 10 seconds. Place noodles, other toppings, fresh cilantro, and a sqeeze of lime juice in the centre of the paper, then begin rolling by folding the two ends inside and continuing to roll encasing all of the ingredients into a tight wrap.

4. Arrange on a platter and serve with the sweet chili sauce for dipping.

Note from the Kitchen:

Make three of these rolls as a light meal or serve as a crowd-pleasing appetizer or delicious snack! If preparing these ahead of time or for lunches, wrap each roll with a damp paper towel to keep the rice paper from drying out and tearing.

Note about Digestion:

If using a hot pepper, note that the more seeds you use, the more heat there will be! Very spicy foods can cause digestive upset so this may be something you should avoid.

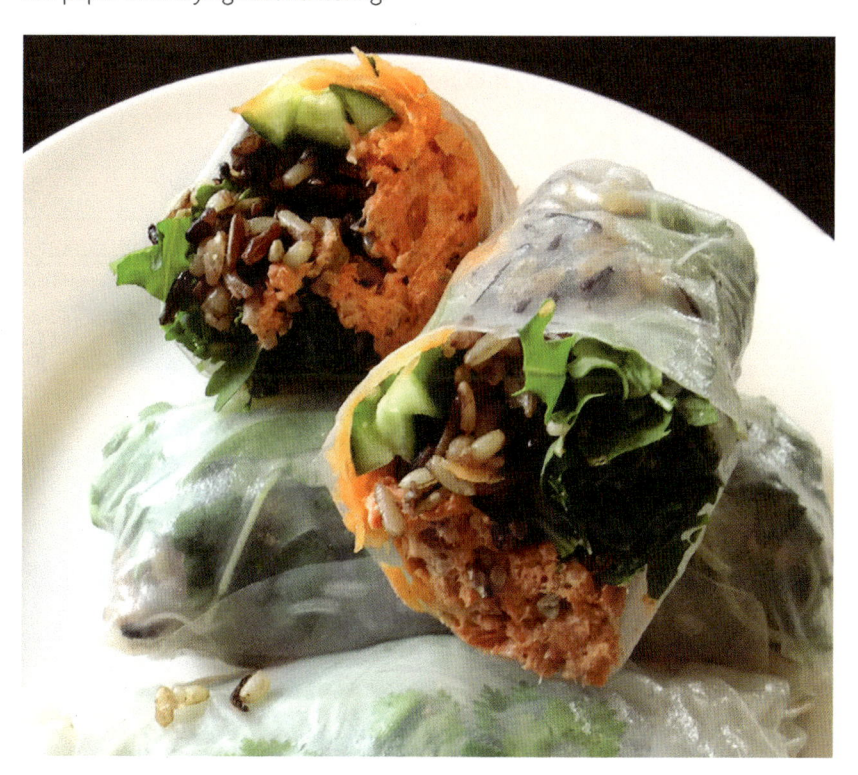

Spanish Quinoa Side Salad

Makes 2 servings

Prep time: 5 minutes

INGREDIENTS

1 ½ cups cooked quinoa

1 celery stalk, diced small

¼ to ½ jalapeno, diced small, or more or less to taste

½ cup cherry tomatoes, halved

¼ cup roasted red peppers, diced small

1 green onion, diced (green part only)

Dash of EACH—chili pepper, paprika, cumin, coriander

Juice of ½ to 1 lime

½ tbsp good quality olive oil

½ tbsp walnut oil

Fresh cilantro

INSTRUCTIONS

1. Combine all ingredients in a large bowl and toss gently to coat. Refrigerate for at least 30 minutes if possible to allow flavours to mingle, otherwise serve immediately. Add more dressing as needed.

Protein Power Side Salad

Makes 4 servings

Prep time: 5 minutes

INGREDIENTS

4 cups baby spinach or other baby mixed greens

1 cup tomatoes, diced

½ cup cucumber, diced

1 medium carrot, grated

½ cup canned chickpeas, drained and rinsed

2 tbsp chia seeds

2 tbsp hulled hemp seeds

Dressing

2 tbsp fresh sqeezed orange juice

1 tbsp olive oil

1 tbsp apple cider vinegar

1 tsp maple syrup

INSTRUCTIONS

1. Arrange greens in a salad bowl or platter and top with the tomatoes, cucumber, grated carrot, chickpeas, chia seeds, and hemp seeds.
2. Whisk together ingredients for dressing in a bowl and drizzle over the top of salad before serving.

Lemon Arugula Side Salad

Makes 4 servings

Prep time: 5 minutes

INGREDIENTS

4 cups arugula, preferably local and organic

1 tbsp good quality olive oil

1 tbsp fresh squeezed lemon juice

Pinch of white sugar

Salt and pepper to taste

2 tbsp pine nuts

Freshly grated Parmesan cheese

INSTRUCTIONS

1. Arrange arugula in a large salad bowl or plate. Whisk together the olive oil, lemon juice, sugar, salt, and pepper and drizzle over the arugula. Top with the pine nuts and parmesan cheese and serve immediately.

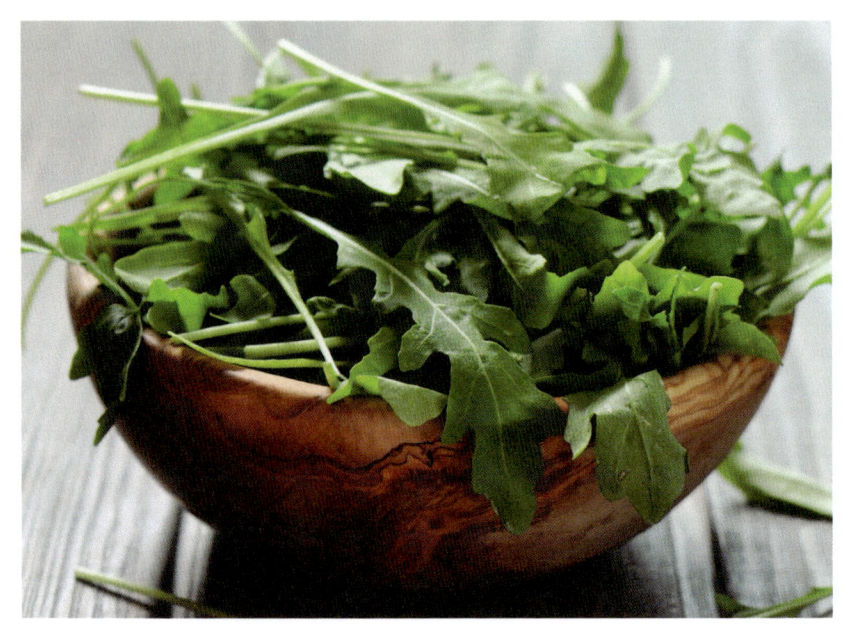

Caprese Side Salad

Makes 4 servings

Prep time: 5 minutes

INGREDIENTS

4 cups baby spinach

1 cup sliced tomatoes (any variety)

1 tbsp good quality olive oil

1 tbsp good quality balsamic vinegar

Salt and pepper to taste

Fresh basil leaves, torn in half

1 oz fresh mozzarella or Buffalo mozzarella each
*If not a symptom trigger

INSTRUCTIONS

1. Place spinach in a salad bowl or on a platter and top with the sliced tomatoes.
2. Whisk together the olive oil, vinegar, salt, and pepper. Drizzle over the spinach and tomatoes and top with the fresh basil. Slice the mozzarella and add on top. Serve immediately.

Note about Digestion:

Leave out fresh or Buffalo mozzarella if the FODMAP lactose is a trigger for you. Try other kinds of cheese like sliced regular mozzarella, crumbled feta, or an aged cheese like Grana Padano or Parmesan.

Spring Pea Risotto

Makes 4 servings

Prep time: 5 minutes | Cook time: 20 minutes

INGREDIENTS

4 cups vegetable or chicken stock

4 cups of water

1 cup fresh peas

2 tbsp olive oil

½ cup fennel pieces, cut into small dice

1 cup Arborio rice

½ cup white wine

½ tbsp butter or GF, LF margarine (like Earth Balance or Becel brand)

4 cups baby spinach leaves

Salt and pepper to taste

Fresh lemon and Grana Padano cheese, to serve.

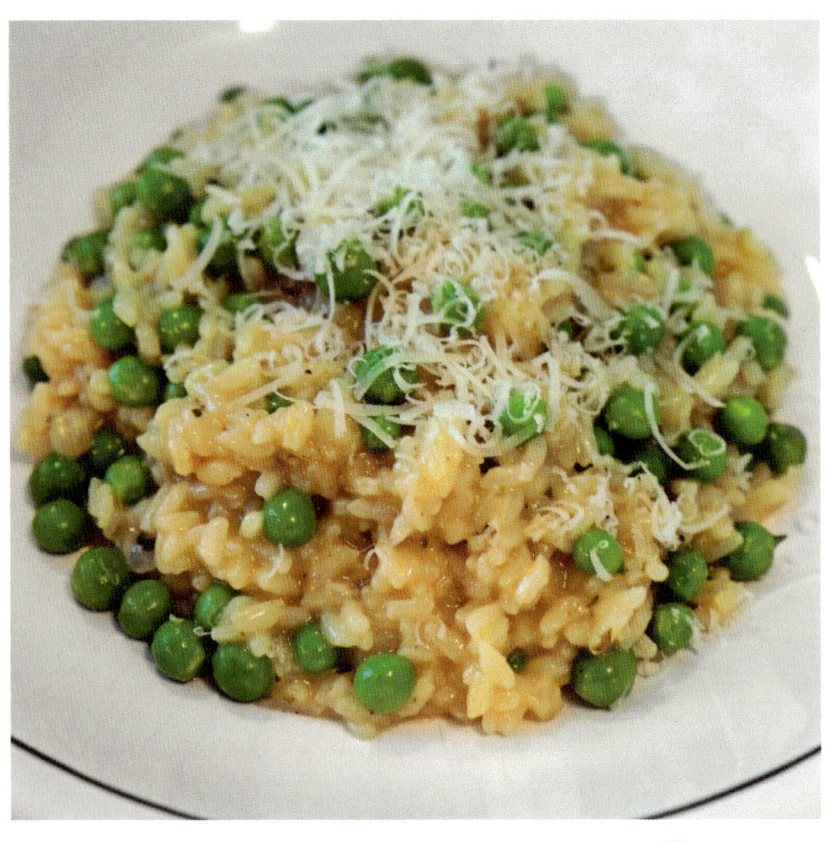

INSTRUCTIONS

1. Heat stock and water in a small saucepan and bring to a simmer. Cover and allow to simmer at the very lowest of settings during the whole recipe. Add peas to simmering stock and cook just 2 to 4 minutes or until tender. Remove with a slotted spoon and place in an ice bath (bowl of cold water with ice) to stop the cooking.

2. In a large, heavy-bottomed metal pot heat the olive oil on medium. Add the fennel and sauté 3 to 5 minutes, until slightly softened. Add the rice and stir so that each grain is coated in oil. Add white wine and reduce for 1 to 2 minutes or until nearly evaporated. Season with a little salt and pepper.

3. Turn the heat to medium-high. Add hot stock, one ladle at a time, while continuously stirring. Allow the rice to absorb all of the stock so that as you stir the pot the bottom is sticky and there is little to no liquid remaining. Add another ladle of stock. Again allow the rice to absorb all the stock. After 3 to 4 ladles of stock, turn down the heat to medium. You may add stock more generously, and you do not have to reduce down all of the liquid before the next ladle of stock. (You can put your spoon down for 30 seconds at a time now and allow the risotto to cook, but don't walk away too far.)

4. About halfway through cooking, about 10 to 12 minutes, add the butter or Earth Balance (or olive oil). Somewhere between 18 and 23 minutes, your risotto will be the perfect texture. You may not need all of the stock—keep tasting it during this time. The risotto is done when the rice is soft, but still a little firm (al dente). Add your peas one minute before your risotto is done, then stir in the spinach until wilted.

5. Serve with a fresh squeeze of lemon and a little Grana Padano or Parmesan cheese. Season with additional salt and pepper to taste.

Note about Digestion:

Grana Padano and other aged cheeses are very low in lactose, some sources estimate 0.1% lactose. These cheeses are generally acceptable on a low FODMAP and lactose-free diet. Green peas are high in the FODMAP oligos in servings over ¼ cup, so if this is a trigger food for you, ensure you stick to the serving size here in the recipe.

Grilled Vegetables and Potatoes

Makes 4 servings

Prep time: 10 minutes | Cook time: 10 to 20 minutes

INGREDIENTS

4 cups small new or red potatoes

2 red, yellow, or orange bell peppers

2 medium yellow zucchini

Olive oil

Salt and pepper to taste

Fresh rosemary, minced

INSTRUCTIONS

1. Preheat the BBQ or grill.
2. Slice the potatoes in half, prick with a fork and cook in the microwave for 4 to 5 minutes until nearly tender. Alternatively, you can parboil potatoes in a large pot of boiling water for 3 to 5 minutes. Meanwhile, quarter the bell peppers and slice the zucchini about 1 cm thick. Rub with a little olive oil, salt, and pepper. Set aside.
3. Rub the potatoes with olive oil and season with salt, pepper, and rosemary. Place on the hot grill skin side up. Add the peppers and zucchini to the grill. Be mindful of hot spots on your BBQ/grill and remove vegetables as they are done. Some may cook faster than others depending on several factors, like size, heat, hot spots, how often you flip and rotate, etc. Grill until vegetables are nicely grill marked and tender throughout.
4. Serve alongside roasted chicken, grilled fish, or any other meat or meat alternative you wish.

Note from the Kitchen:

This grill recipe works great for other low FODMAP vegetables as well like sweet potato (½ cup per person), eggplant, squash, or parsnips. Instead of using a BBQ, alternatively you could grill vegetables on your stove top using an iron skillet or grill pan.

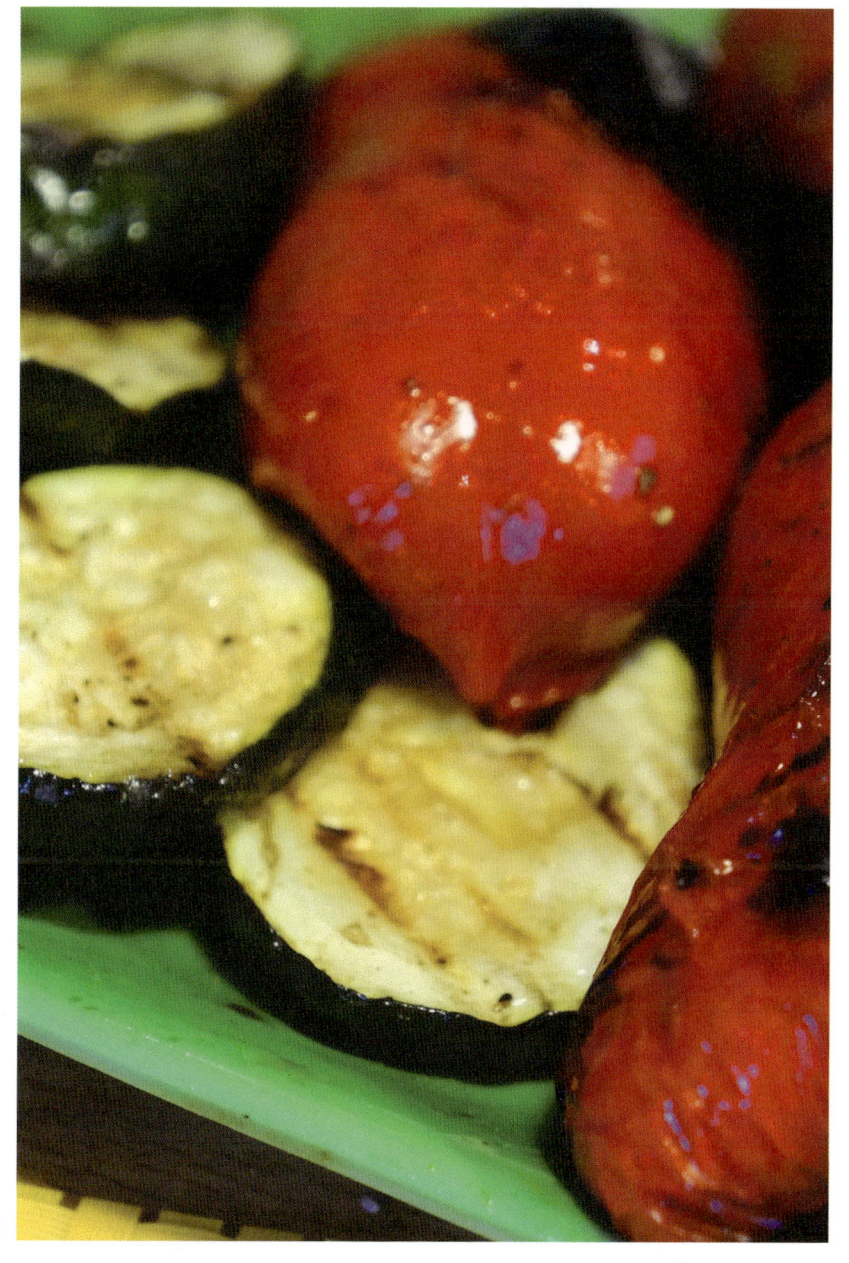

Meatless Meals

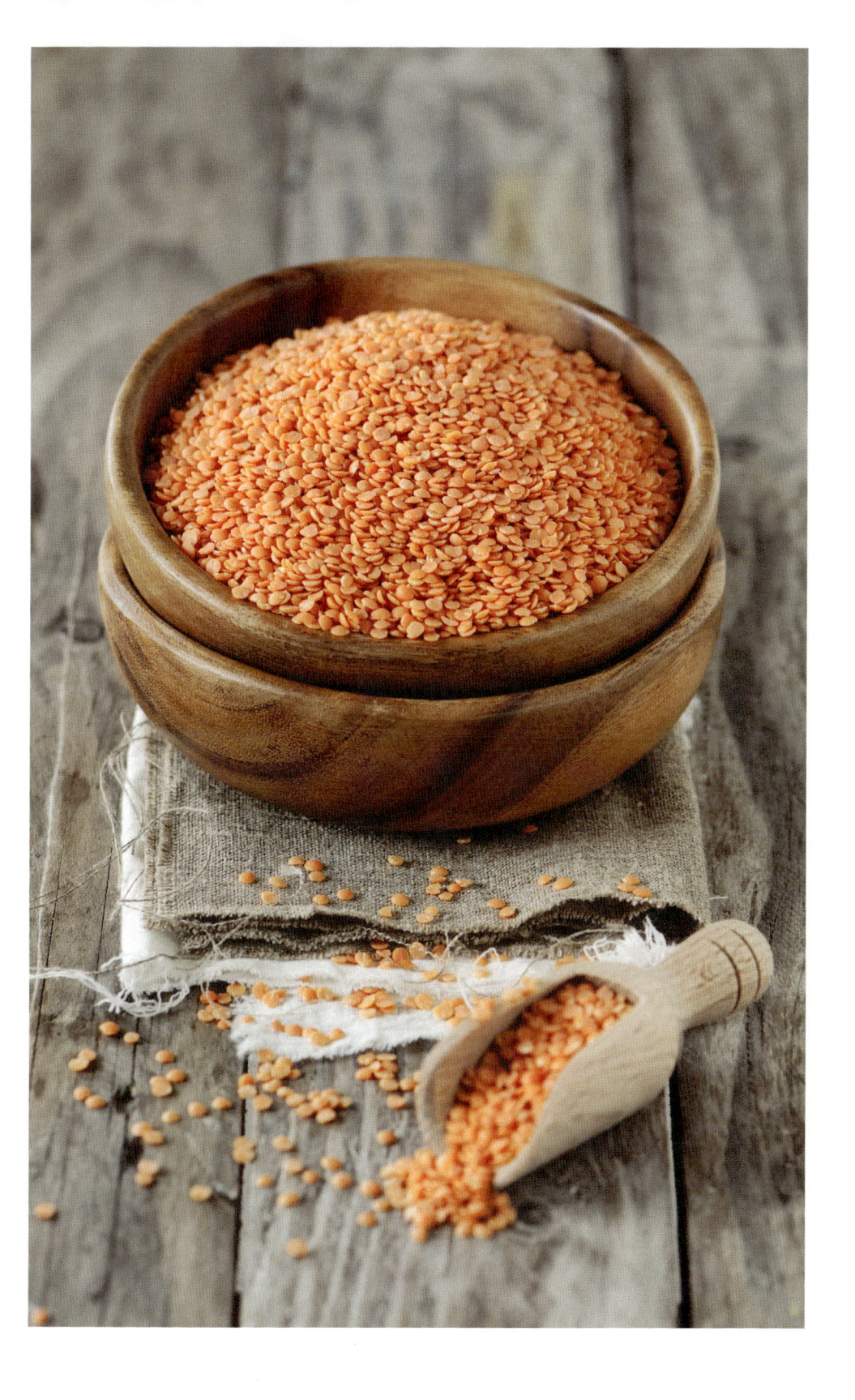

Vegetarian Vegetable Bolognese

Makes 4 servings

Prep time: 20 minutes | Cook time: 35-40 minutes

INGREDIENTS

Tempeh (2 blocks), crumbled OR substitute 1 lb ground lean beef, chicken, or turkey

1 tbsp olive oil

¼ cup red wine *optional

½ cup fennel, diced

2 stalks celery, diced

1 large (about 1 cup) carrot, diced

1 red and 1 yellow bell pepper, diced

1 can pureed tomatoes, preferable local brand (i.e., Ontario Natural) or passata

1 tsp EACH dried parsley, thyme, oregano, and basil

½ lb dry gluten-free pasta i.e. spaghetti, penne, or rigatoni (about 4 to 5 cups cooked)

4 cups spinach, chopped

INSTRUCTIONS

1. If using the tempeh, place in a small pot of boiling water for 10 minutes. This step allows some of the fermented flavour to release. Remove from water and let the tempeh cool for 5 minutes before crumbling. Dry with a paper towel before moving to the next step.

2. Heat a large, metal pot on medium-high heat. Add 1 tbsp olive oil. Add crumbled tempeh, beef, chicken, or turkey. Allow to stick to pan. Cook until brown, flipping only when tempeh or meat releases from the pan, about 5 to 6 minutes. Once cooked, add ¼ cup wine or water to deglaze, scraping up the little brown bits. Remove tempeh or meat from pan and set aside.

3. Reduce heat to medium-low and add olive oil. Add fennel, celery, and carrot. Cook for 5 minutes. Add peppers and cook for 5 minutes more. Add tempeh or meat back to pot along with tomatoes, parsley, thyme, oregano, and basil. Bring to a boil, reduce heat, and simmer for 20 minutes.

4. Meanwhile cook your pasta according to package directions.

5. Turn off heat and stir in spinach. Serve with pasta.

Note from the Kitchen:

My favourite brand of gluten-free pasta is La Venezianne. It's made with corn from Italy and tastes as beautiful as classic Italian white pasta. One package or ½ lb of pasta will serve four people.

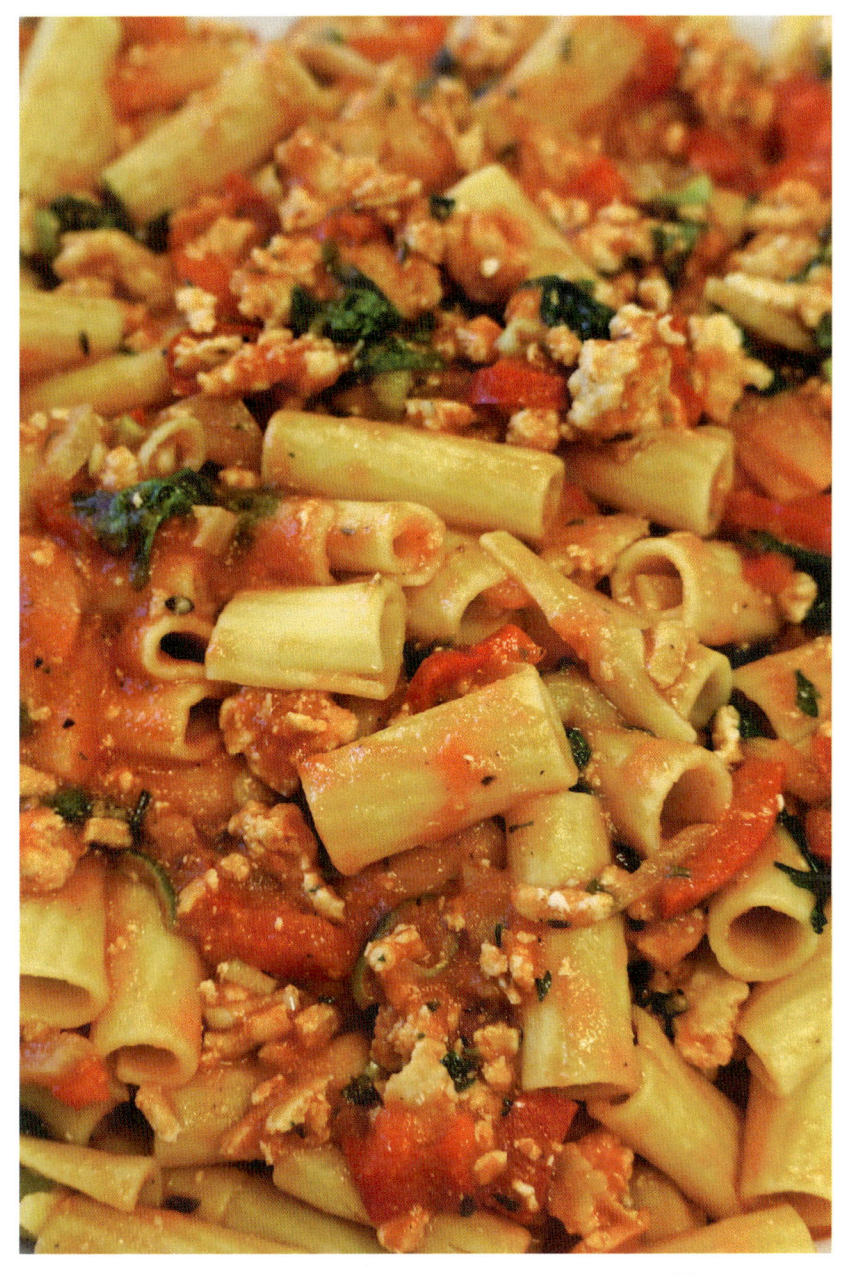

Smokey Tempeh and Lentil Chili

Makes 4 servings

Prep time: 15 minutes | Cook time: 55 minutes

INGREDIENTS

1 tbsp olive oil

1 block tempeh, crumbled (alternatively ½ lbs ground chicken, turkey, or lean beef instead, if desired)

2 tsp chili powder

¼ tsp EACH cumin, parsley, smoked paprika, and chili flakes

Dash cayenne pepper

½ cup red wine

1 tbsp olive oil

½ cup fennel, diced

1 stalk celery, diced

1 cup carrots, sliced thin

1 yellow pepper, diced

1 can (750 mL) crushed (preferrably roasted) tomatoes

1 tbsp maple syrup

½ tsp liquid smoke

1 tsp tamari (gluten free)

1 cup canned lentils

INSTRUCTIONS

1. Heat a metal skillet on medium heat. Add 1 tbsp olive oil and crumbled tempeh. Allow the tempeh to stick to the pan to brown, about 2 to 3 minutes. Add cumin, parsley, paprika, chili, cayenne, salt and pepper and stir. Cook 2 to 3 minutes more until browned then add the wine to deglaze the pan. Remove tempeh from pan, but keep the pan on medium heat.

2. Add 1 tbsp olive oil, fennel, celery, carrot, and pepper to the hot pan. Sauté 5 minutes. Add tempeh back into pan. Add tomatoes, maple syrup, liquid smoke, tamari, and lentils. Bring to a boil, partially cover and let simmer for 45 minutes.

3. Serve with homemade GF corn bread (or Bob's Red Mill variety) or GF toast.

Note from the Kitchen:

This recipe can also be prepared in a crockpot. Follow step 1 to brown the tempeh and then add all ingredients to a crockpot. Cook on low for 8 hours.

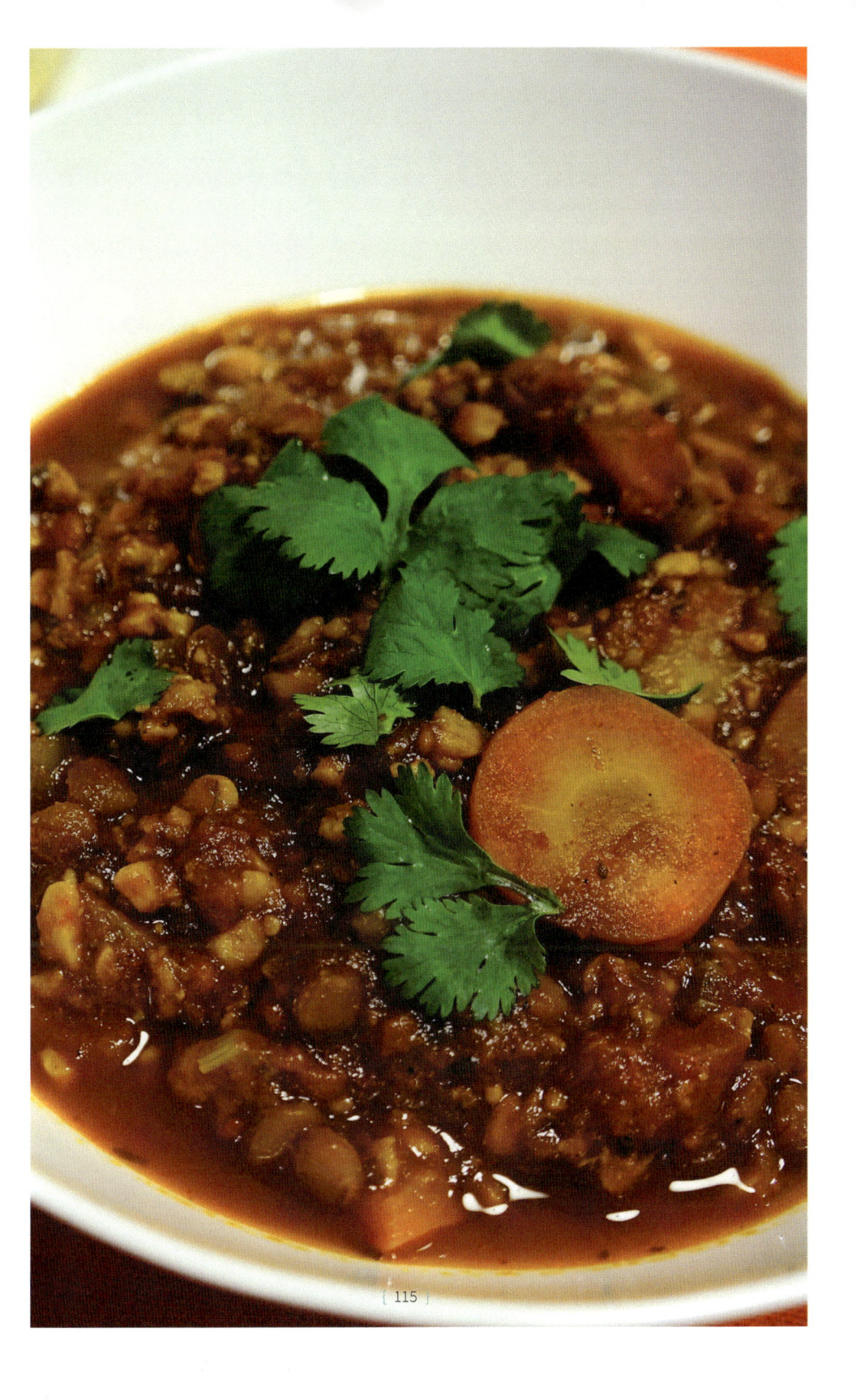

Spinach Salad Bowls with Tempeh Bacon

Makes 4 servings

Prep time: 10 minutes | Cook time: 20 minutes

INGREDIENTS

For the bowl

2 medium sweet potatoes (about 2 cups)

1 tsp olive oil

4 cups baby spinach or other mixed baby greens

1 large carrot, peeled and grated

½ medium cucumber, diced small

¼ cup sesame seeds

For tempeh bacon

1 block organic tempeh (about 250 g)

1 tbsp liquid smoke

1 tbsp tamari (gluten-free)

1 tbsp sesame oil

1 tbsp olive oil

1 tbsp apple cider vinegar

1 tbsp maple syrup

Pinch of granulated garlic and/or onion powder
*If not a symptom trigger

For the dressing

2 tbsp sesame oil

1 tbsp rice vinegar

1 tbsp maple syrup

Juice of ½ lemon

Salt and pepper to taste

INSTRUCTIONS

1. Preheat the oven to 425°F.

2. Cut sweet potatoes into quarters, prick with a fork, and place in a microwave safe bowl. Cook in microwave for 4 to 5 minutes or until nearly tender. Toss with the olive oil, salt, and pepper and place on a lined baking sheet. Complete cooking in the oven for about 10-15 minutes until browned and crispy.

3. Slice tempeh width-wise into 20 thin strips (about 3 mm thick). Mix together the tempeh ingredients in a small bowl and coat each strip with the sauce. Place on the same lined baking sheet used for the potato and broil on high (500°F) for 3 to 6 minutes per side until golden brown and crispy. (Be mindful to not overcook the tempeh as it can burn very easily.) In a small bowl stir together the dressing ingredients.

4. To serve, toss together the spinach and dressing, transfer to a platter and top with the carrots, cucumbers, tempeh bacon, sweet potato, and sesame seeds.

Note from the Kitchen:

Try a variety of proteins in this dish like chicken, ground pork, shrimp, tofu, nuts, or seeds.

Note about Digestion:

Sweet potato in large servings is high in the FODMAP polyols (sugar alcohols). If this is a trigger food for you, ensure you do not consume more than ½ cup as outlined in this recipe and be mindful, even this small amount may be a trigger for digestive symptoms.

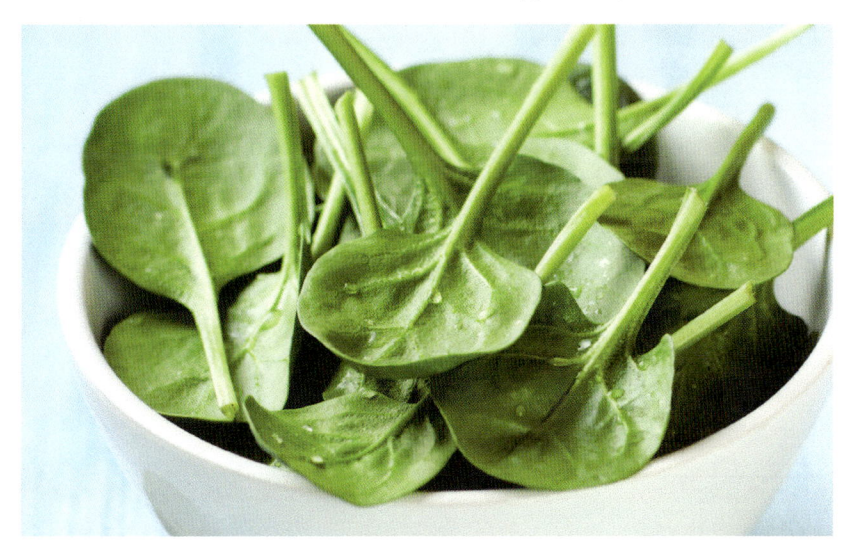

Tempeh Taco Salad

Makes 4 servings

Prep time: 10 minutes | Cook time: 20 minutes

INGREDIENTS

1 block of tempeh (about 250 g)

1 cup quinoa, uncooked

¼ cup of white wine or vegetable stock

6 cups of seasonal, leafy greens like Boston lettuce, baby spinach, or mixed greens

2 cups cherry tomatoes, diced

1 cup cucumber, diced

Fresh cilantro

½ an avocado, peeled, seeded, and diced small

¼ cup grated old cheddar cheese

Handful of gluten-free nacho chips

1 tbsp olive oil

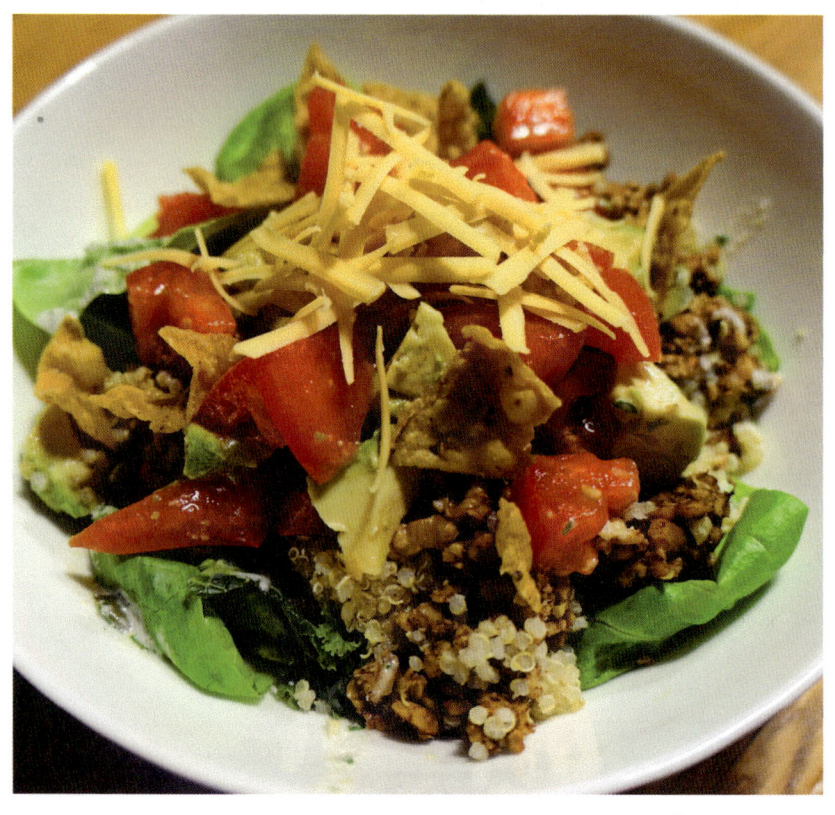

Seasoning

2 tsp chili powder

1 tsp ground coriander

½ tsp cumin

½ tsp smoked paprika

¼ cup walnuts, crumbled

Dressing

4 tbsp fresh orange juice

2 tbsp olive oil

2 tbsp apple cider vinegar

1 tbsp maple syrup

Salt and pepper

INSTRUCTIONS

1. Bring a small pot of water to a boil. Place block of tempeh in the boiling water and cook 10 minutes. Remove, place in a colander and break tempeh into pieces. Allow to cool and drain. Rinse quinoa. Place into a small pot with 1 ½ cups of water. Bring to a boil, cover and simmer 15 minutes until tender.

2. In a small bowl stir together the seasoning ingredients. Once tempeh has cooled slightly, crumble into small pieces and place in a medium bowl with the seasoning mix. Toss to coat.

3. Add the olive oil to a large metal sauté pan on medium heat. Add tempeh and brown by spreading out evenly in the hot metal pan without stirring or flipping. Allow it to stick to the pan to cause actually brown colouring on the pan. Stir once browning has begun, cooking for 3 to 5 minutes. Add a little white wine or stock to pan to deglaze, scraping up all the little brown bits of flavour stuck to the pan. Remove from heat.

4. To serve, toss the greens, tomatoes, cucumber, and cilantro with a little of the dressing provided or a simple dressing with low FODMAP ingredients. Top with the cooked tempeh, avocado, cheese, quinoa, and nacho chips.

Note from the Kitchen:

Use this recipe to make delicious wraps, leave out the quinoa and chips. Add the tempeh mixture to corn tortillas and top with greens, tomato, cilantro, avocado, and cheese.

Crunchy Cornmeal-Crusted Tofu in Collard Wraps with Quinoa

Makes 4 servings

Prep time: 1 hour | Cook time: 15 minutes

INGREDIENTS

Tofu and marinade

2 tbsp tamari (gluten free)

1 tbsp maple syrup

1 tbsp sesame oil

Juice of 1 lime

½ tsp cumin

½ tsp ground coriander

1 large block or 2 small blocks (450 g) firm tofu, preferably organic

1–2 tbsp olive oil

Cornmeal Coating

½ cup cornmeal

½ tsp chili pepper

½ tsp red pepper flakes OR Epicure 5 pepper blend

½ tsp cayenne

Chipotle mayo

¼ cup veganaise or mayonnaise

Juice of ¼ lime

½ tsp dried oregano

Pinch of cayenne

1 diced chipotle pepper in adobo sauce

To Serve

8 large collard leaves

2 cups cooked quinoa

1 red or yellow bell pepper, sliced

½ cucumber, diced

INSTRUCTIONS

1. Make tofu marinade by combining tamari, maple syrup, sesame oil, lime juice, cumin and coriander in a shallow bowl or dish. Slice tofu across to make 2 large rectangles (about ¾ to 1 cm thick); then slice into four squares and slice the squares diagonally to make triangular pieces. You should have about 16 pieces. Place tofu in marinade and soak for one hour, flipping once.

2. Meanwhile, combine all ingredients for cornmeal coating in a bowl or dish and set aside. Combine all ingredients for the chipotle mayo and set aside (in the fridge).

3. Once tofu has marinated, heat a large non-stick skillet on medium heat with a little of the olive oil. Coat each piece of tofu in the cornmeal coating by tossing gently in the mixture and pressing firmly to stick, shaking off excess. Place in the skillet, making sure to hear a sizzle, indicating the oil is hot enough. Cook for 2 to 4 minutes per side until browned and crispy.

4. To serve spread a little mayo on a large collard leaf. Place 2 to 4 tbsp quinoa, bell peppers, cucumber, and the tofu on top. Finish with a little more mayo as desired and wrap up.

Note from the Kitchen:

Use a small brownie pan or large flat-bottomed bowl to marinade your tofu. Substitute or add in other vegetables to wrap as desired—like grated carrots, sprouts, etc.

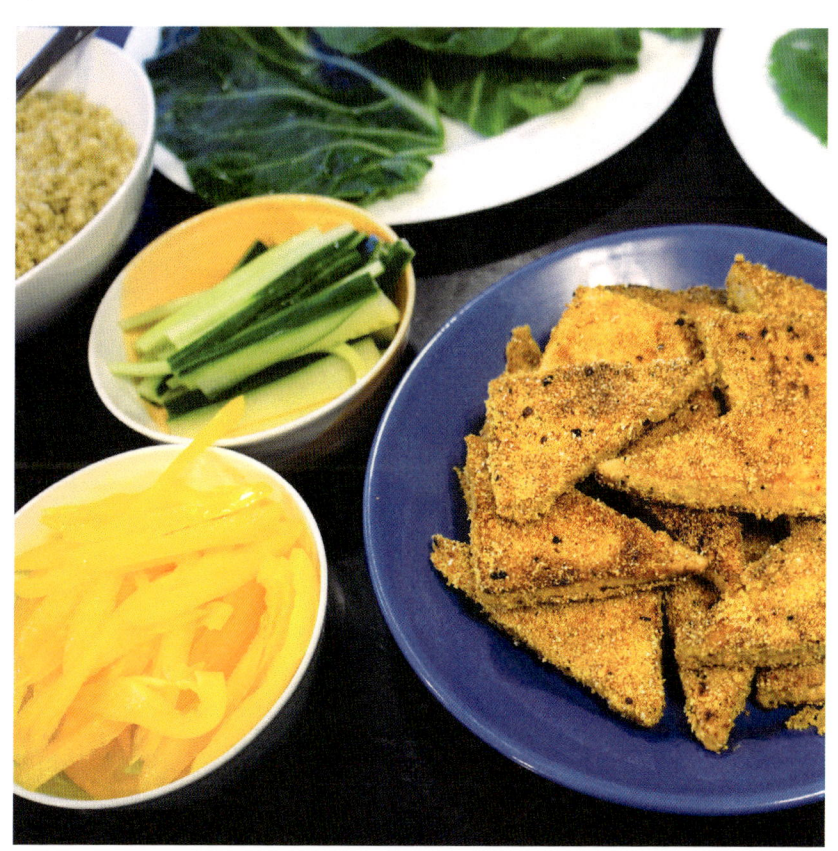

Easy Lentil Quesadillas

Makes 4 servings

Prep time: 15 minutes | Cook time: 5 minutes

INGREDIENTS

1 ½ cups canned lentils OR substitute for cooked chicken, shrimp, or beef (2–3 oz per person)

½ avocado

Seasoning as desired like cayenne, 5 pepper blend, cajun, chili powder, cumin, OR onion and garlic powder if tolerated

Freshly ground pepper and salt to taste

4 large gluten-free tortillas like Food for Life, Udi's, or La Tortilla Factory Teff wraps

Handful of fresh cilantro, chopped

1 cup bell peppers, cherry tomatoes, spinach, or other desired vegetable topping, diced small

*Optional: grated OLD cheddar cheese or other well-tolerated cheese

1 tsp olive oil

INSTRUCTIONS

1. Warm tortillas in the microwave for 30 to 45 seconds or in the oven wrapped in tinfoil so they do not dry out.

2. Combine lentils, avocado, and seasoning in a flat-bottomed bowl. Mash with a 'potato masher' until ingredients are combined. If using chicken, shrimp, or beef simply mix ingredients together. Spread mixture evenly on one-half of each of the tortillas.

3. Meanwhile, heat olive oil in a large non-stick pan.

4. Top the filling with vegetables of choice being careful not to make quesadilla too thick. Fold in half and if using cheese place this side up.

5. Cook 2 minutes per side in the hot oil until crunchy and golden. Serve with a handful of salad, mixed greens, or cooked vegetables.

Note about Digestion:

Beans and lentils can be very difficult to digest for many. This recipe uses a small amount of lentils as they are easiest on digestion of all the pulses. The serving here is slightly high in FODMAPs and may be challenging for some. If so, use ground chicken, tempeh, beef, or a combination of lentils and one of these ingredients.

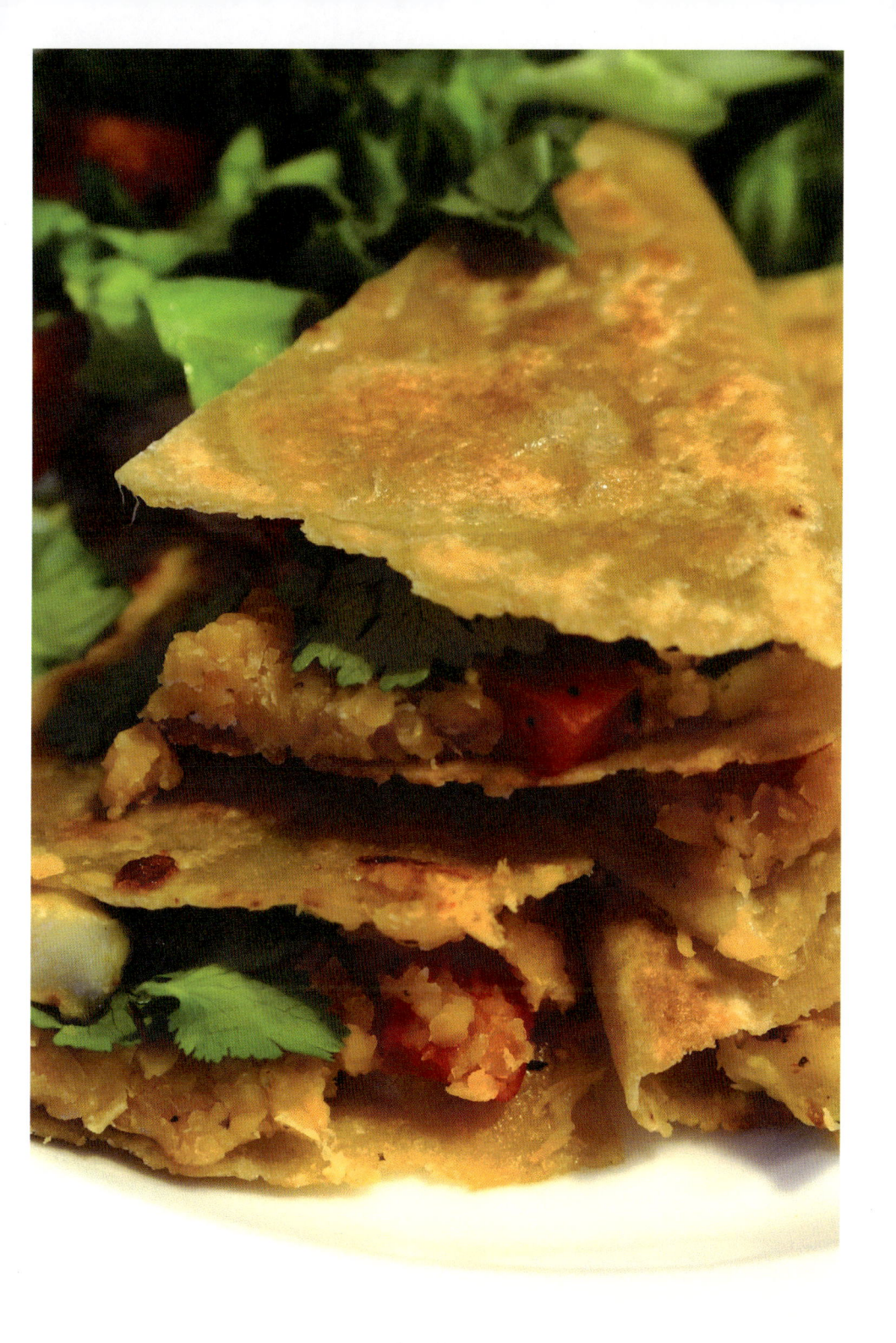

Pan-Fried Cod with Vegetable Quinoa

Fish tastes best when it's fresh. Ask your local fish monger for the freshest catch. Fish shouldn't smell or taste fishy if it's fresh. Enjoy this simple recipe with fresh and meaty cod.

Makes 4 servings

Prep time: 10 minutes | Cook time: 20-25 minutes

INGREDIENTS

- 2 cups quinoa
- Olive oil
- ¼ tsp chili flakes
- 1 medium eggplant (3 to 4 cups), diced medium
- 3 red bell peppers (3 to 4 cups), diced medium
- 1 tsp EACH dried oregano, parsley, and basil
- Salt and pepper
- 1 ½ lbs of fresh boneless, skinless cod, cut into four portions
- Handful fresh parsley, finely chopped
- Fresh lemon

INSTRUCTIONS

1. Rinse quinoa and add to a medium sauce pan with 3 cups of water. Cover, bring to a boil, reduce heat and simmer for 15 minutes. Once cooked remove the lid and fluff with a fork. Set aside.

2. Meanwhile, place a metal skillet on medium heat. Add 2 tbsp olive oil and chili flakes. After one minute add eggplant, oregano, parsley, basil, and cook 5 minutes. Add bell pepper and cook 5 minutes more. Eggplant should be cooked through and the pepper tender but still crisp.

3. Once vegetables are cooked, add to quinoa along with the juice of half a lemon. Season with salt and pepper to taste, cover and keep warm.

4. Warm a non-stick skillet on medium heat. Add 1 tsp olive oil and place cod pieces on the skillet. Allow to brown, about 2 to 3 minutes per side and flip over. Once cooked, serve with vegetable and quinoa mixture. Top with more olive oil, fresh parsley and lemon as desired.

Note from the Kitchen:

If fresh cod is not available from your fish market, alternatively you can use pickerel, tilapia, or haddock.

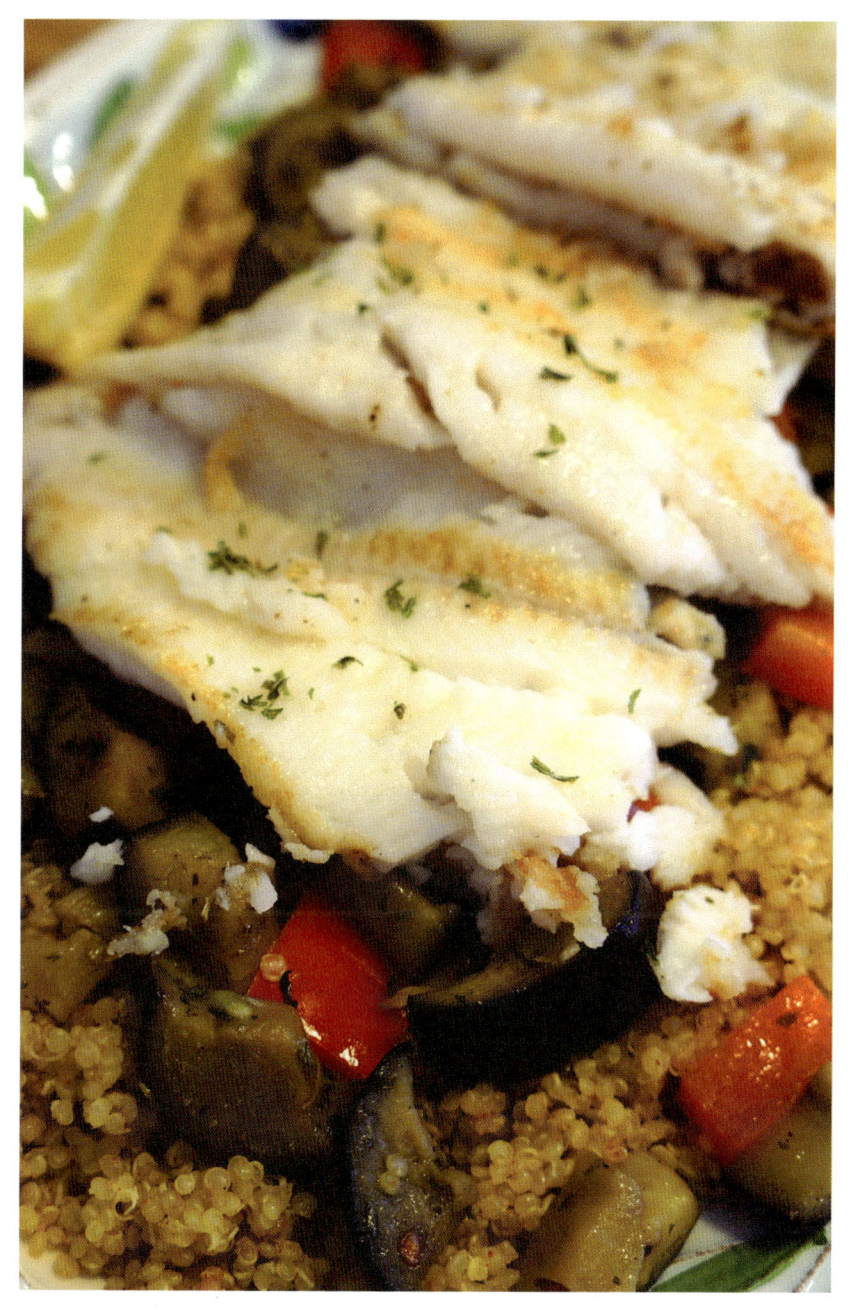

Breaded Cod with Rice Pilaf

Makes 4 servings

Prep time: 10 minutes | Cook time: 20 minutes

INGREDIENTS

1 tsp olive oil

½ cup fennel, diced small

½ cup carrot, diced small

2 stalks celery, diced small

1 cup jasmine or basmati rice

¼ cup white wine

1 ¼ cups water or stock

1 bay leaf

Zest of 1 lemon

1 ½ lbs fresh boneless, skinless cod, cut into four portions

Freshly ground pepper and a pinch of salt

⅛ cup white rice flour

1 large egg, beaten

½ cup gluten-free breadcrumbs

1 tsp parsley

1 tsp olive oil

INSTRUCTIONS

5. Make the rice pilaf by heating the olive oil in a small metal pot on medium heat. Add the fennel, carrot, and celery and cook 4 to 6 minutes until soft and translucent. Add rice and stir until each grain is coated with oil. Add wine and cook for a few seconds until almost all the liquid is gone. Add water or stock, bay leaf, and zest, place lid on the pot and bring to a boil. Reduce heat to low and cook 20 minutes until tender or according to package directions. Remove from heat.

6. Meanwhile, season the fish with salt and pepper and set aside. Place rice flour, egg, and breadcrumbs each in their own shallow bowl. Mix the parsley with breadcrumbs.

7. Heat a large non-stick pan on medium heat with the olive oil. One at a time, toss each of the pieces of fish in the flour, gently shaking off excess. Using the other hand, coat fish with egg and then place in breadcrumbs, pressing the crumbs into the fish. Place each piece of fish in the hot pan so that you hear the sizzle. (If you don't hear the sizzle, turn up the heat and wait for the pan to get warm enough before adding the fish.) Cook 2 to 4 minutes per side depending on the thickness of the fish, until golden brown and inside is white.

8. Serve immediately with rice pilaf and a side of grilled vegetables, sautéed green beans, or salad for a complete meal.

Note about Digestion:

Instead of the fennel, you can use shallots, which are small, sweet onions but are high in the FODMAP oligos. If this is not a symptom trigger for you, opt to use the shallot instead to build flavour.

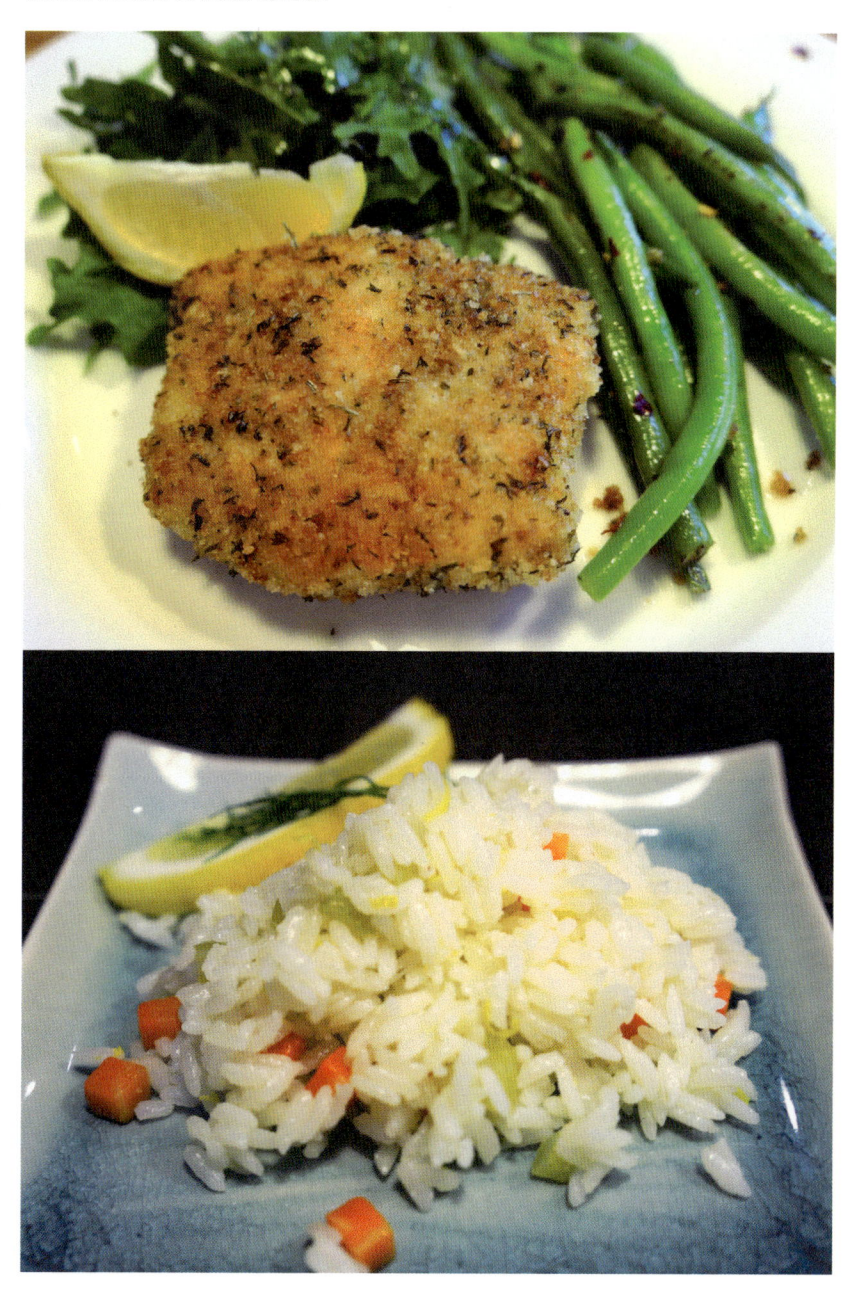

Grilled Pickerel

A simple way to prepare fish is to buy the freshest catch, sprinkle a little salt and pepper or other seasoning on top, and grill on an iron grill pan on your stove or on the BBQ. It's simple and delicious. Here's my favourite local Ontario version.

Makes 4 servings

Prep time: 2 minutes | Cook time: 10 minutes

INGREDIENTS

1 ½ lbs fresh pickerel, cut into four portions

2 tsp olive oil

Freshly ground pepper and a pinch of salt

Pinch EACH of cumin, coriander, paprika, and cayenne (just enough to sprinkle)

Fresh lemon slices

INSTRUCTIONS

1. Place a large iron grill pan on medium heat. Alternatively, heat your grill or BBQ to medium high.
2. Rub the fish with olive oil and season with salt and pepper. Add just a light sprinkle of each spice (or more if you like it spicy!).
3. Place each piece of fish on the hot grill. Cook 3 to 4 minutes per side depending on the thickness of the fish, until grill lines form and the inside is white and solid.
4. Serve immediately with a starch and vegetable.

Note from the Kitchen:

Pair this dish with the Spanish Quinoa Side Salad for a perfectly balanced (and delicious) meal.

Note about Digestion:

Instead of the fennel, you can use shallots, which are small, sweet onions but high in the FODMAP oligos. If this is not a symptom trigger for you, opt to use the shallot instead to build flavour.

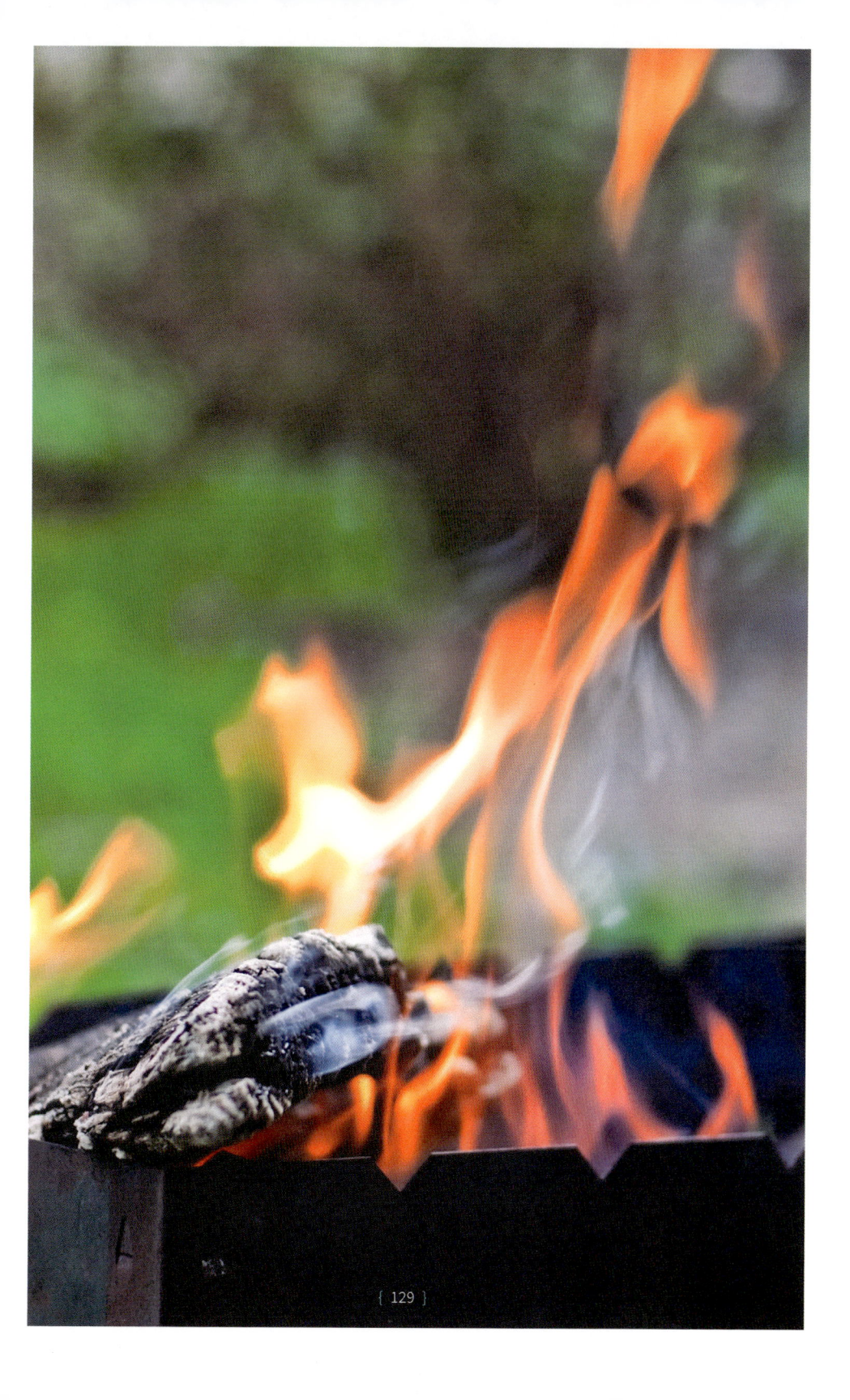

Salmon en Papillotte

Makes 4 servings

Prep time: 10 minutes | Cook time: 15 to 18 minutes

INGREDIENTS

1 ½ cups white, brown, or wild rice blend (preferably Lundsberg brand)

2 red or yellow bell peppers, sliced thinly

2 cups green beans, trimmed

1 cup fennel, chopped into large pieces

1 tsp olive oil

Salt and pepper

1 ½ lbs salmon, cut into four portions

4 cloves of garlic (for flavour, not for eating)

A couple shallots, quartered OR whole green onions (for flavour, not for eating)

Handful of fresh dill

2 limes, sliced into rounds

Olive oil

White wine *optional

INSTRUCTIONS

1. Preheat oven to 400°F.
2. Bring 2 to 3 cups of water to a boil (depending on package directions) in a medium pot. Add rice. Cover, reduce heat, simmer and cook according to package directions (about 20 to 50 minutes, depending on the type of rice).
3. Meanwhile, cut 4 large pieces of parchment paper OR use 4 parchment paper pockets/bags.
4. Toss pepper, beans, and fennel in olive oil. Season with salt and pepper.
5. Place the salmon, skin side down in the middle of the parchment paper. Place the peppers, beans, and fennel to one side of the salmon. Place the garlic, shallots or green onions, dill, and lime on top of the salmon. Drizzle a little olive oil and white wine if desired. Season with more salt and pepper.
6. Fold paper around the edges to make a pocket, ensuring that no air can escape. Place on a cookie sheet and bake for 12 to 18 minutes, until cooked through.
7. To serve, make a long cut on top of pouch to let steam out. Serve with ½ to 1 cup rice.

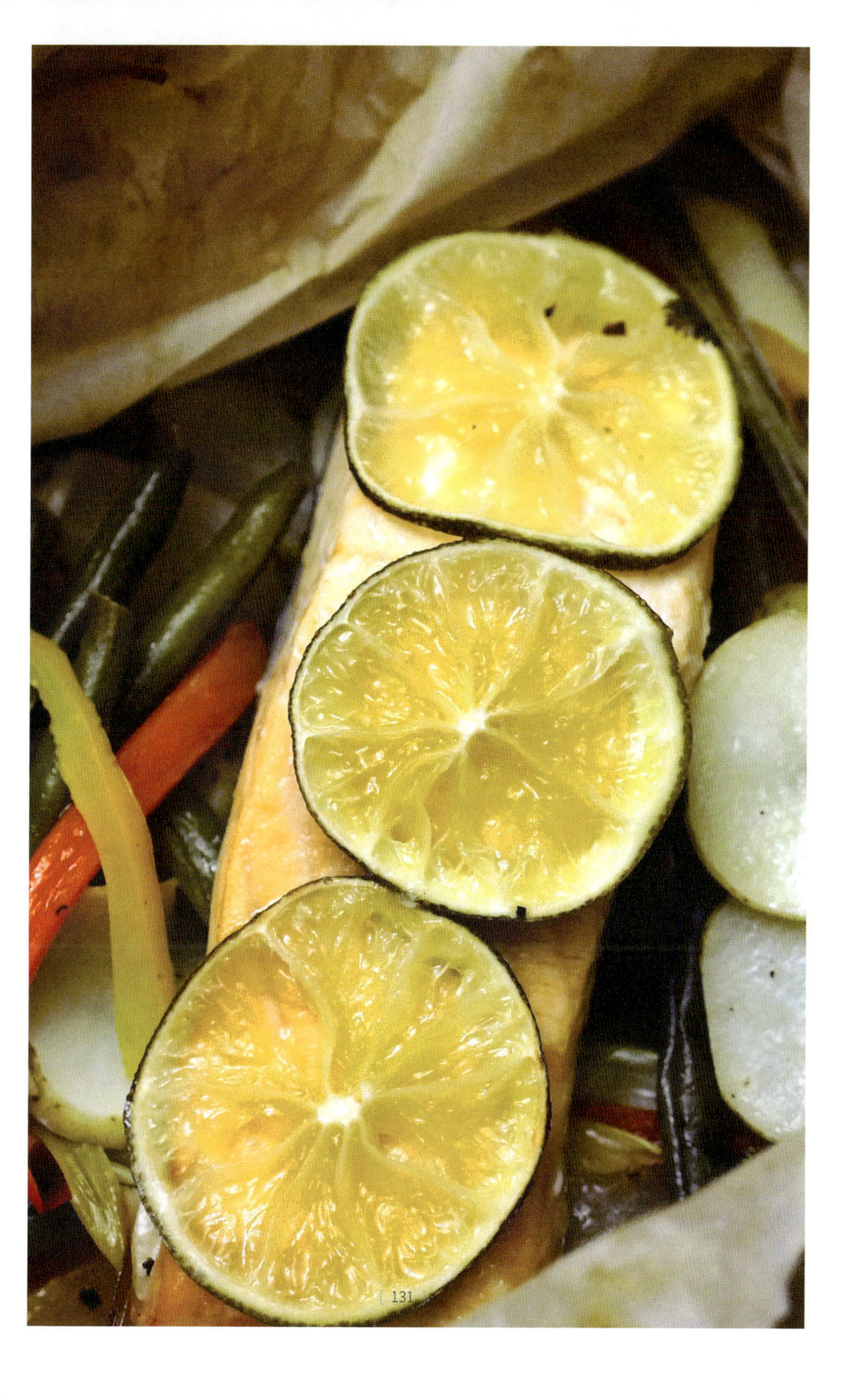

Salmon Kale Salad Sandwiches

Makes 4 servings

Prep time: 5 minutes | Cook time: 5 minutes

INGREDIENTS

1 lb cooked salmon, leftover or cooked fresh

¼ cup (2 large) green onions, minced (green part only)

¼ cup (4 large leaves) kale, minced

4 GF buns or toasted baguette (try Udi's crusty baguettes)

½ cup grated carrots

½ cup cucumber, diced

Sauce

2 tbsp lemon juice (about ½ lemon)

2 tbsp mayonnaise

1 tbsp plain lactose-free yogurt

1 tsp Dijon mustard

2 tbsp fresh parsley, minced

¼ tsp dried thyme

Salt and pepper to taste

INSTRUCTIONS

1. Using a fork, flake salmon in to small pieces. Place in a large bowl with green onion and kale.

2. In a separate bowl, add sauce ingredients and whisk together. Add the sauce to the salmon and combine.

3. Serve one-quarter of the salmon, carrots, and cucumber in your bun and serve with a salad.

Note from the Kitchen

If using fresh salmon for this recipe, cut into four pieces and bake at 425°F for 10 to 15 minutes, until cooked through. Allow to cool for a few minutes before flaking. This salmon kale salad can be enjoyed any way you please from topped on a crustini as an appetizer to scooped on a salad. My favourite way to enjoy this recipe is by taking about 1/12 of the mixture along with a couple tablespoons of cooked rice and adding grated vegetables like carrots and cucumbers to a moistened rice paper. Roll it up and serve three as a perfect lunch, dinner, or as an amazing appetizer. You'll love it!

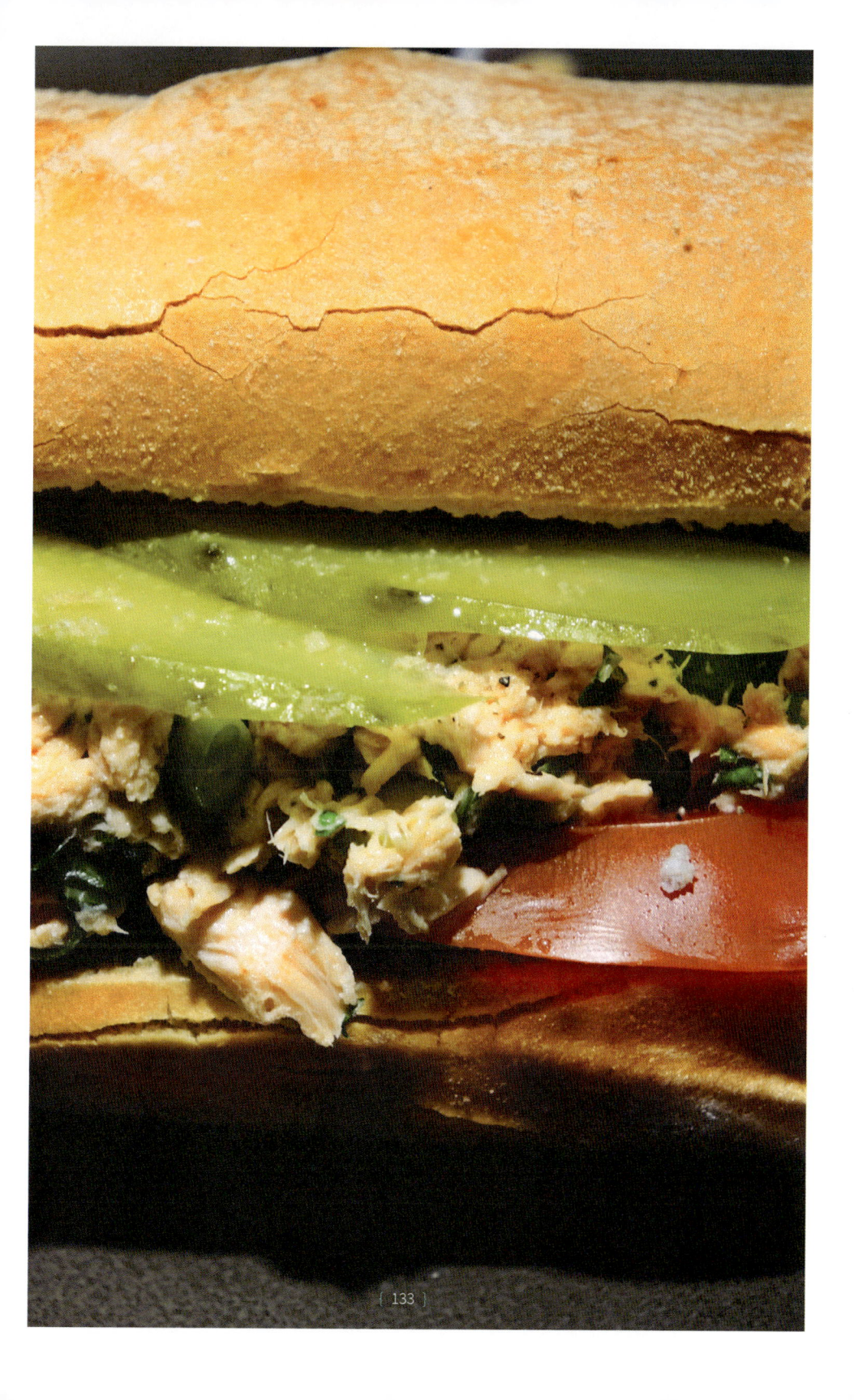

Corn-Crusted Trout

Makes 4 servings

Prep time: 10 minutes | Cook time: 25–30 minutes

INGREDIENTS

1 ½ lbs of fresh trout, cut into four portions

¼ cup corn flour

For the vegetables

4 cups potatoes, washed and cubed	Pinch of salt and freshly ground pepper	3 (3 to 4 cups) red peppers, diced
Olive oil	1 cup fennel, diced	1 tbsp sesame oil
1 tsp EACH dried sage, oregano, and parsley	3 cups green beans, trimmed and diced	2 tbsp sliced almonds
		Juice of 1 lemon

INSTRUCTIONS

1. Preheat oven to 425°F.
2. Place chopped potatoes in a glass dish and microwave on high for 5 minutes. Toss in oil, sage, oregano, parsley, and a little salt and pepper. Place on a baking sheet and put into the oven.
3. Meanwhile, heat a skillet on medium heat and add 1 tbsp olive oil. Add fennel and sauté 5 minutes. Add green beans and red pepper. Sauté 5 minutes more. Once cooked to tender but still crisp, remove from heat and top with sesame oil, almonds, and lemon juice. Set aside and keep warm.
4. Season trout with salt and pepper if desired. Toss in corn flour and gently shake off excess.
5. Warm a non-stick skillet on medium heat with 1 tsp of olive oil. Add fish, skin side down, and cook 5 minutes. Flip and continue to cook until the fish is still moist but cooked through—about 2 to 4 minutes more.
6. Serve with potatoes and vegetables.

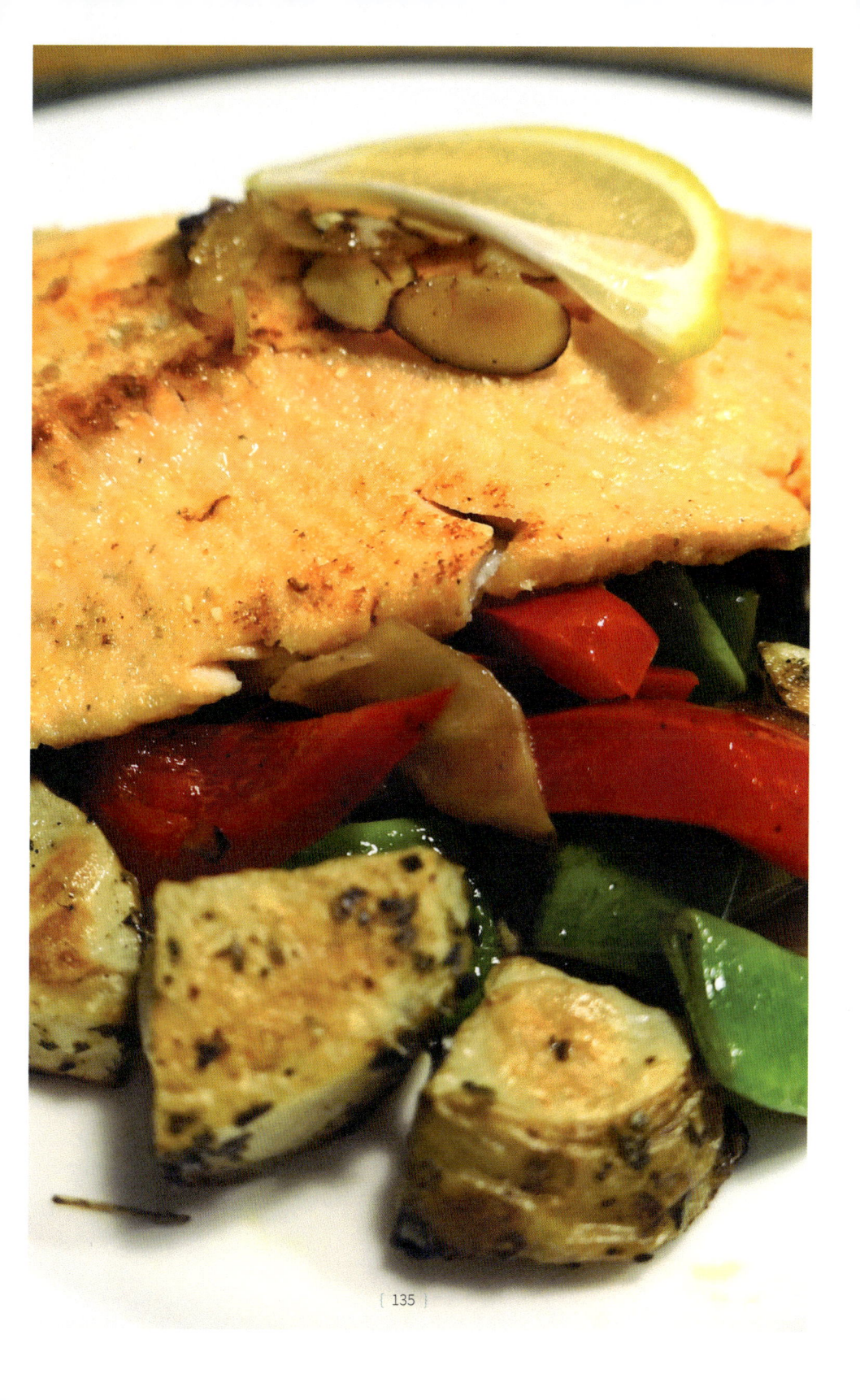

Roasted Red Pepper Tuna Quinoa Cakes

Makes 4 servings (8 to 12 cakes total)

Prep time: 5 minutes | Cook time: 8 minutes

INGREDIENTS

2 cans flaked tuna, in water, preferably sustainably caught, drained

2 green onions, diced (green parts only)

1 ½ cups cooked quinoa, preferably 1 day old

1 large roasted red pepper, diced very small

1 large egg

1 tbsp veganaise or mayonnaise

½ tsp Dijon mustard

Juice of 1 lemon

½ tsp dried cilantro

½ tsp dried parsley

⅛ tsp salt

Freshly ground pepper

½ cup gluten-free breadcrumbs

Olive oil, preferably in a spray or spritzer

Chipotle mayo, to serve (See recipe on page 120)

INSTRUCTIONS

1. Preheat the oven to 400°F.
2. Add all ingredients except for breadcrumbs and olive oil to a large bowl and mix well. Form into 8 or 12 equally-sized balls and place on a clean flat surface. Using the palm of your hand, gently flatten the balls to about ½ inch thick patties.
3. Spread breadcrumbs onto a flat dish and one-by-one coat the outside of the tuna cakes with breadcrumbs, pressing gently. Place on a non-stick baking sheet OR a regular baking sheet lined with parchment paper. Spray a little bit of olive oil on each side of the tuna cakes. If not using a spritzer, drizzle just a small amount of oil on each side of the patties or use a BBQ or pastry brush to thinly coat.
4. Bake for 20 to 30 minutes or until cakes are brown and the surface is crispy, flipping once during cooking after about 15 minutes. Serve with a little chipotle mayo and a side salad for a balanced meal.

Note from the Kitchen:

For some heat, consider adding 1 tbsp of diced jalapeno peppers or ½ tsp of red pepper flakes or a pinch of cayenne to the patty mixture.

Note about Digestion:

The white part of the green onion is high in the FODMAP oligos. If this is a trigger for you, ensure you follow the recipe by including just the green part of the green onion; if not, than you can add some of the white of the onion as well.

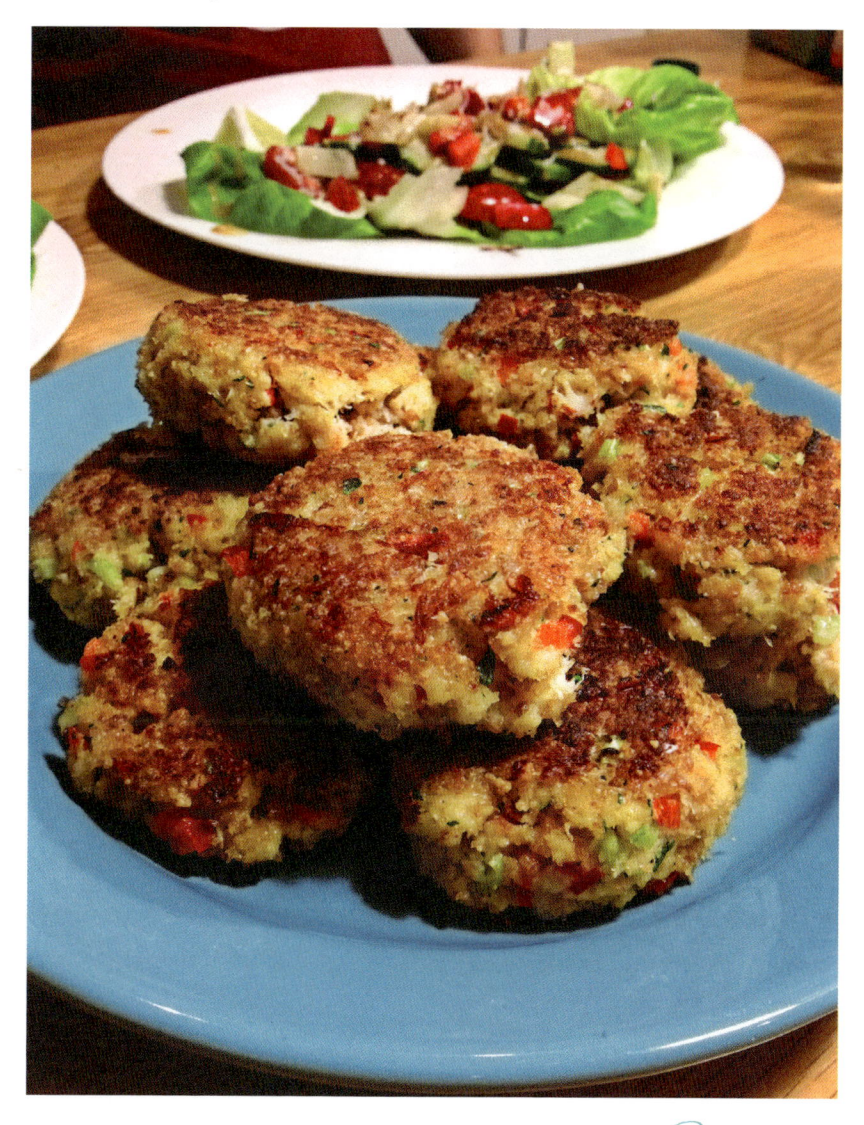

Shrimp Burgers with Tomato Avocado Salsa

Makes 4 servings

Prep time: 15 minutes | Cook time: 10 minutes

INGREDIENTS

1 ½ lbs shrimp, shelled and deveined
(the vein runs along the back of the shrimp), as local as possible

⅓ of a red chili minced OR ¼ tsp chili flakes
(if using fresh chili, remove the seeds if you do not like it too hot)

2 tbsp fresh cilantro, chopped	**For the salsa**
⅛ tsp ground ginger	1 large tomato, diced small
⅛ tsp dried cumin	½ avocado, diced into small pieces
⅛ tsp dried coriander	Juice of ½ a lime
Pinch of salt and freshly ground pepper	1 to 2 green onions, sliced (green part only)
Juice of ½ a lime	Salt and pepper
4 gluten-free buns or 8 slices of gluten-free bread	Garlic-infused olive oil for grilling

INSTRUCTIONS

1. Dice half of the shrimp into ½ inch thick pieces and place in a bowl. Take the other half of the shrimp and puree in a food processor for 15 to 20 seconds until fairly smooth. Add to the bowl.

2. Add chili, cilantro, ginger, cumin, coriander, salt, pepper, and lime to shrimp. Mix with a spoon until well combined. Form into 4 burger patties. Shrimp burgers will be sticky and wet in consistency.

3. Chill burgers in the fridge while you prepare the salsa. Mix tomato, avocado, lime, green onion, salt, and pepper. Season and adjust ingredients as desired. Prepare side salad at this point as well if serving. Remove burgers from fridge.

4. Heat a flat bottomed iron skillet on medium heat. Add 1 to 2 tsp garlic infused oil to pan. Add burgers to hot pan making sure not to overcrowd (two at a time if necessary). Cook 2 to 3 minutes until golden brown and flip gently with a large spatula. Cook 1 to 2 minutes more on the other side until cooked through. Be careful not to overcook or the burger will dry out.

5. Serve on a bun or bread with salsa and a side salad.

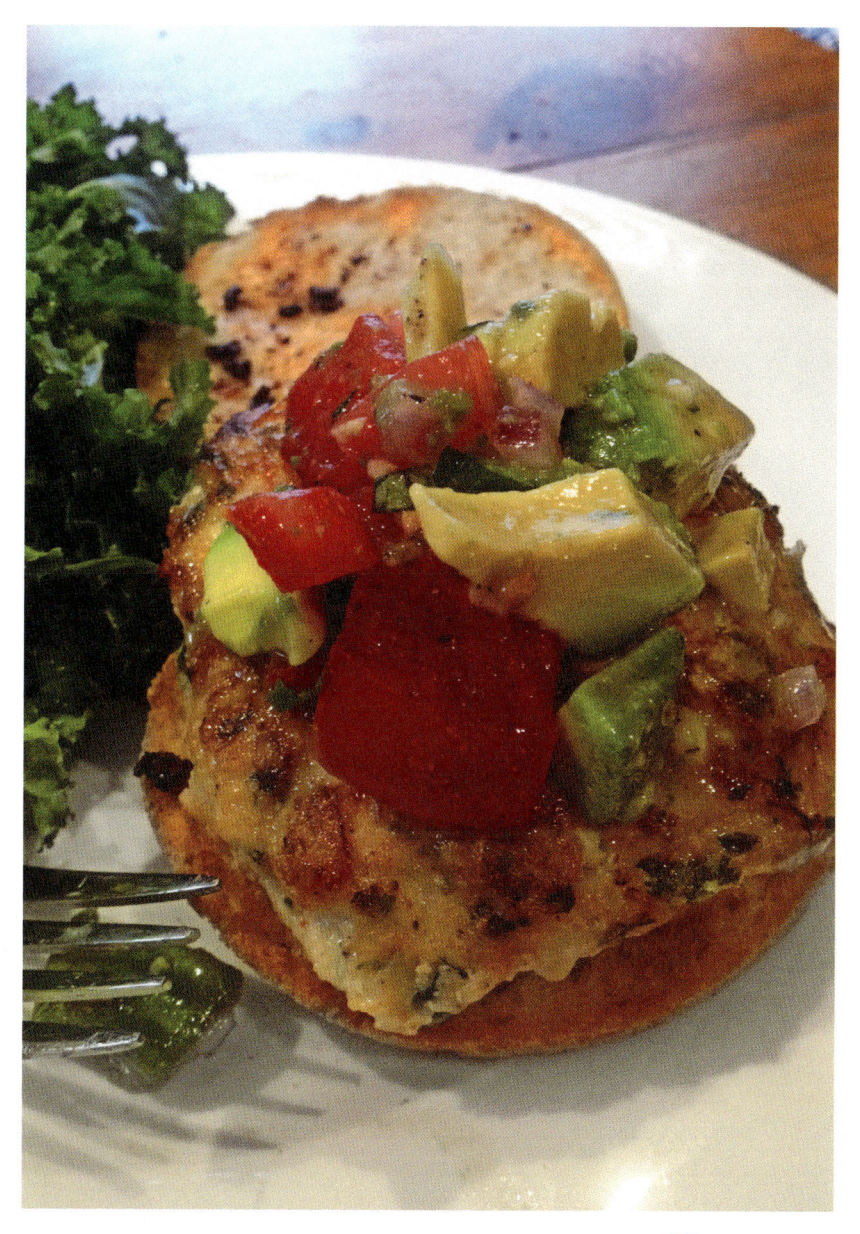

Perfect Peanut Noodle Bowl

Makes 4 servings

Prep time: 15 minutes | Cook time: 45 minutes

INGREDIENTS

For the peanut sauce

2 tbsp sesame oil

1 tbsp tamari (gluten free)

½ tbsp maple syrup

2 tbsp natural, smooth peanut butter

1 tbsp rice vinegar

1 tbsp fresh lime juice

Green onions—green part only, finely chopped

1 tsp grated ginger *optional

For the bowl

1 lb sautéed shrimp or leftover, diced chicken, or tofu prepared the way you like

1 package soba or rice noodles (about 250 to 300 g)

4 to 6 cups fresh or stir-fried vegetables (bell peppers, green beans, cucumbers, radishes, etc.)

2–4 tbsp of sesame or sunflower seeds

INSTRUCTIONS

1. Prepare the shrimp, chicken, or tofu. Consider a quick stir-fry shrimp sautéed in a non-stick pan for 2 minutes per side with a little sesame oil and chili flakes. You can use leftover chicken OR sauté ground chicken in a pan with a little sesame oil, gluten-free tamari, salt, and pepper. Tofu can be marinated in your favourite ingredients (try GF tamari, apple cider vinegar, and sesame oil) and baked until crispy (about 20 minutes).

2. Whisk together sauce ingredients in a blender or with a wire whisk until well-combined. Set aside.

3. Meanwhile, bring a large pot of water to a boil. Add noodles and cook according to package directions.

4. Prepare vegetables by cutting into thin slices.

5. Once noodles are cooked, drain and rinse with hot water. Mix noodles with prepared peanut sauce and place into 4 bowls. Top with vegetables, shrimp, chicken, or tofu, and sprinkle seeds on top as desired. Serve immediately.

Note from the Kitchen:

This recipe is one of my favourites. We have a variation of this almost every week. The recipe is fairly general to allow you to be creative. Try any kind of GF noodle, or rice, or even quinoa for the base of the bowl. Use fresh vegetables or make a quick stir-fry OR use a little raw and a little cooked! This is a great recipe to use up leftover meat, fish, lentils, or tempeh. The sky is the limit here!

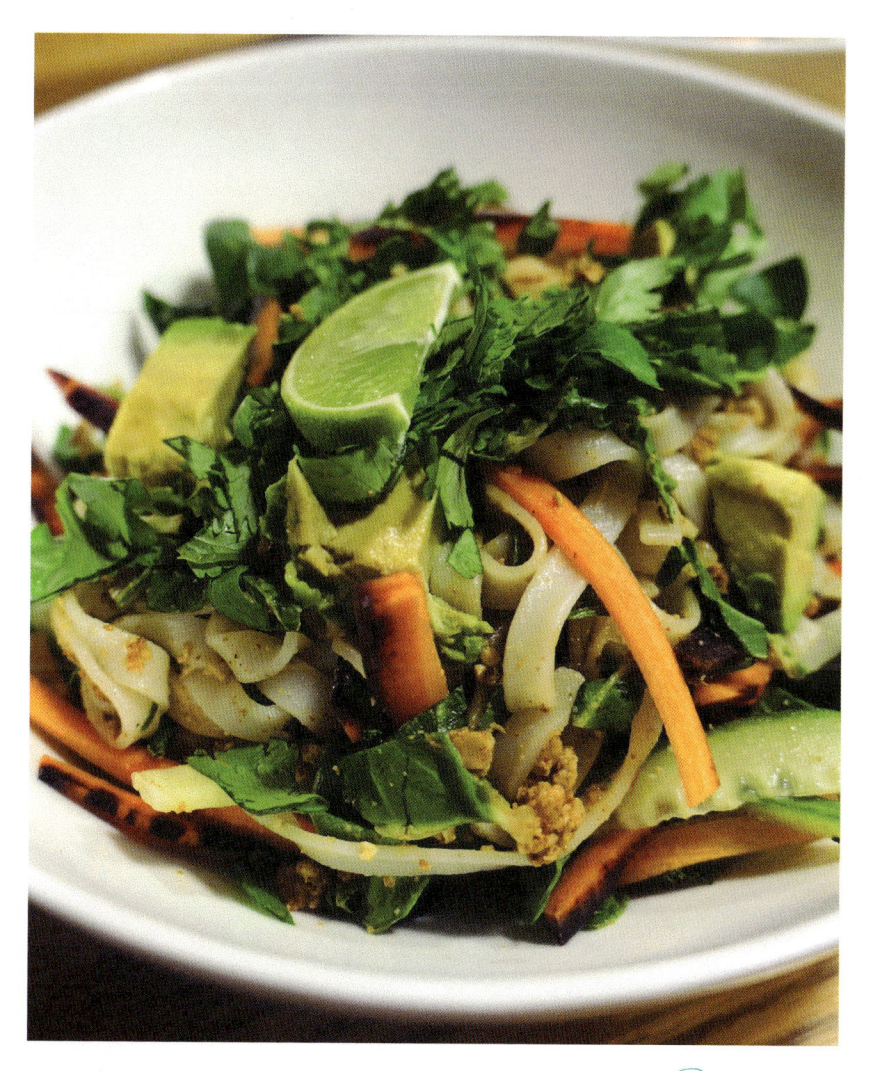

Meat and Poultry

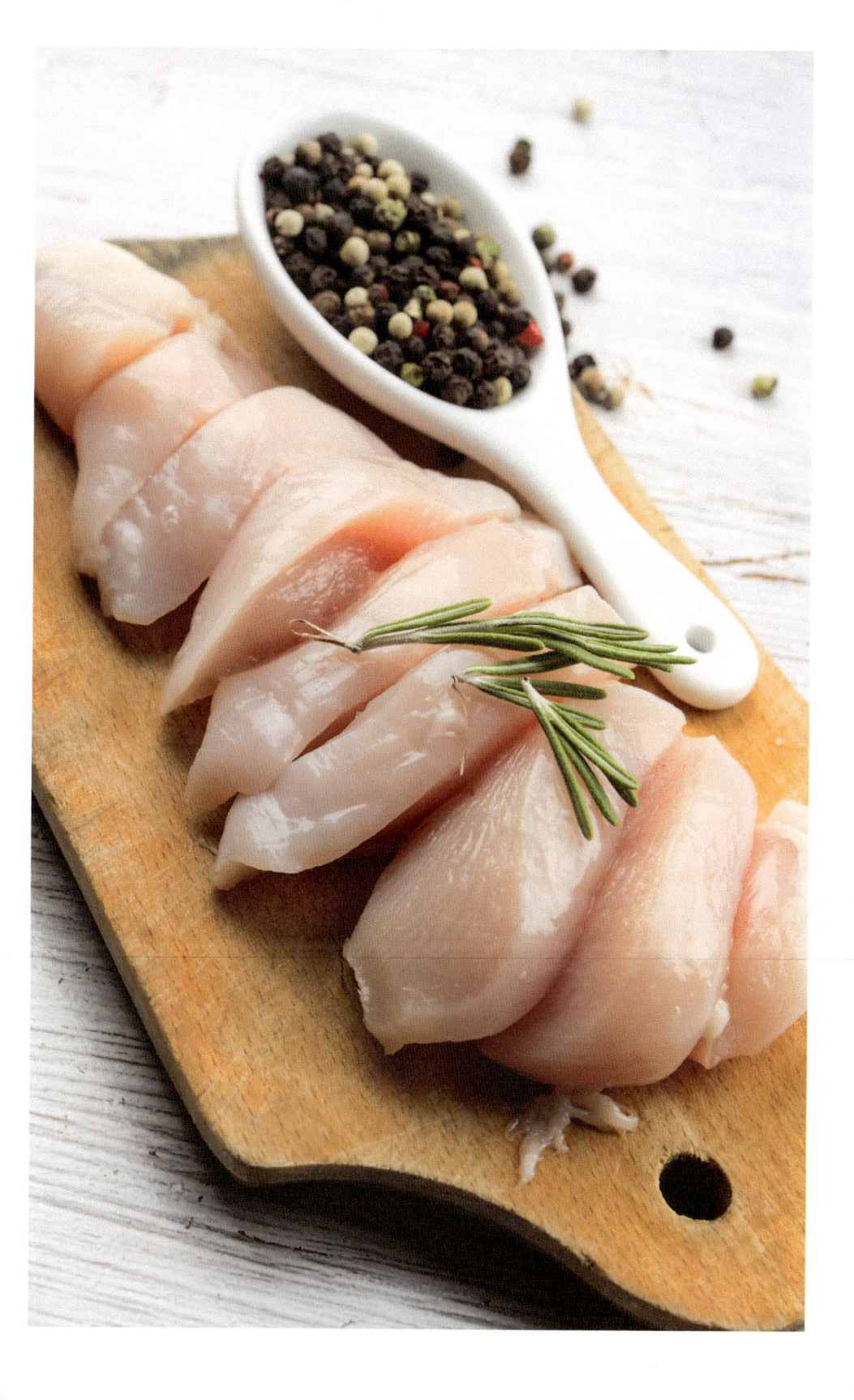

Sesame Chicken Lettuce Tacos with Rice Noodles

Makes 4 servings

Prep time: 10 minutes | Cook time: 20 minutes

INGREDIENTS

1 lb boneless chicken breasts, preferably local and organic

2 tbsp tamari (gluten free)

2 tbsp sesame oil, plus more for noodles

½ pack (about ½ lb) rice vermicelli noodles

1 head Boston lettuce (about 3 to 4 leaves per person)

2 large carrots and/or radishes, shredded

Fresh cilantro

For the sauce

1 tbsp tamari (gluten free)

1 tbsp sesame oil

1 tbsp tahini

Juice of ½ a lime

1 tsp brown sugar

1 green onion, diced (green part only)

INSTRUCTIONS

1. Preheat the oven to 425°F
2. Slice the chicken breast into ½ inch strips. Toss in the tamari and sesame oil, place on a lined baking sheet, and bake for 15 to 20 minutes, until cooked through and lightly browned. (Alternatively, chicken can be grilled, breaded, or pan-fried.)
3. Meanwhile, bring a medium pot of water to a boil. Add rice noodles and cook for 2 to 4 minutes, or according to package directions. Drain and rinse under cool water. Toss in a little sesame oil and set aside, spread out on a dish to cool.
4. In a serving bowl combine the sauce ingredients. Have the lettuce leaves, carrots, and cilantro prepared. To serve, place one strip of chicken on a lettuce leaf with a ¼ cup of noodles, top with the carrots, cilantro, and finish with a little sauce.

Note from the Kitchen:

Use leftover chicken from a meal prior as a time saver! Add a little chili paste or Sriracha sauce to add some heat to your taco. You can also substitute or include other vegetables such as thinly sliced bell pepper or cucumber.

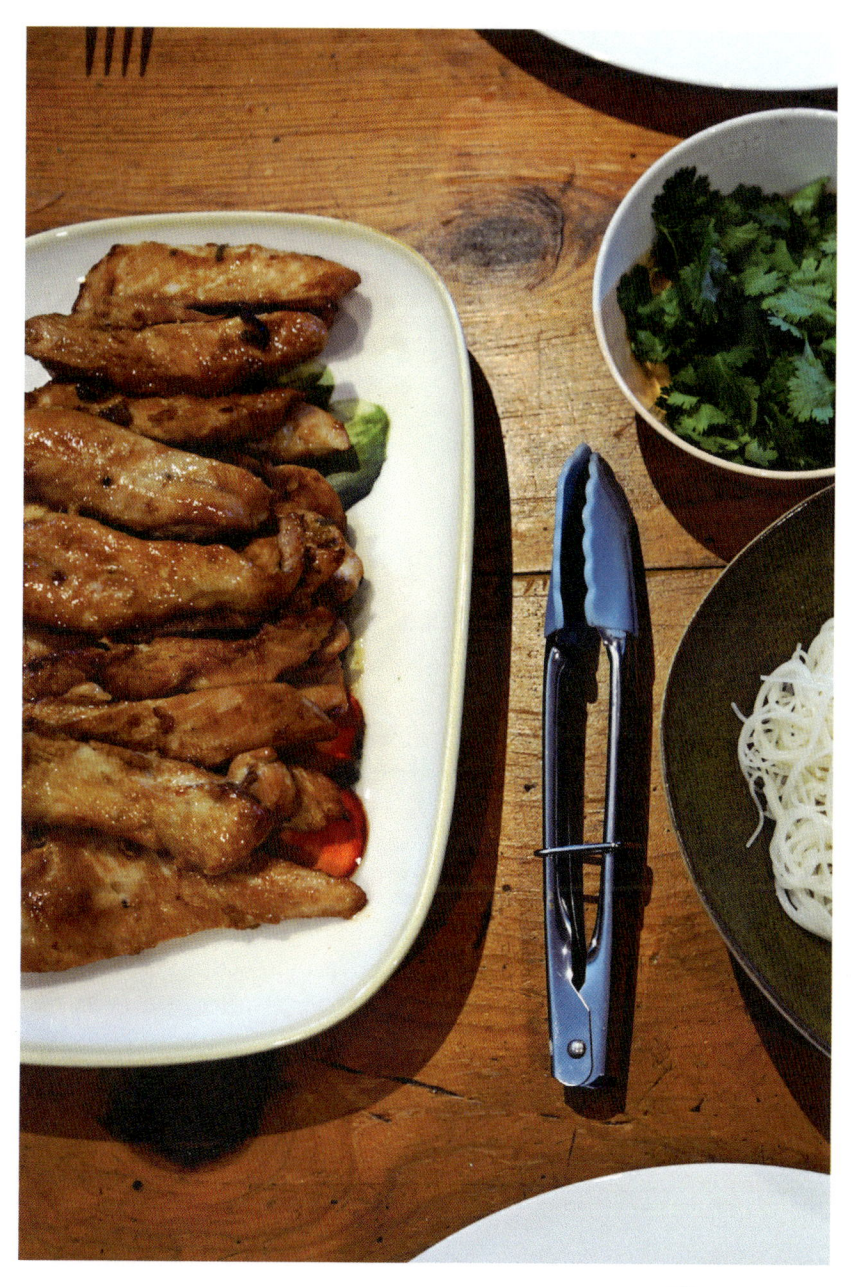

Curry Chicken Salad Lettuce Wraps

Makes 4 servings

Prep time: 10 minutes | Cook time: 15 minutes

INGREDIENTS

500 g chicken breast, boneless, skinless

Salt and pepper

3 tbsp olive oil

½ cup white wine

2 tbsp cider vinegar

1 tbsp maple syrup

½ to 1 tbsp quality curry powder mixture (like S&B brand)

Juice of 1 lime

½ cup fennel, diced small

½ cup red bell pepper, diced small

2 stalks of celery, diced small

2 cups cooked quinoa

Boston lettuce leaves, to serve

INSTRUCTIONS

1. Flatten chicken breasts by slicing in half lengthwise and pounding with a meat mallet. Season with salt and pepper. Heat a large metal skillet on medium to medium-high heat. Add 1 tbsp of olive oil and the chicken, being careful not to overcrowd the pan. Flip after 3 to 4 minutes, once the meat releases from the pan and easily lifts away, while browning. Cook on the other side, until no longer pink inside and nicely browned. Remove from pan, let cool slightly and dice. Set aside.

2. Keep the pan on medium heat and add the wine. Deglaze the pan by scraping at the brown bits. Add chicken back into the pan with remaining olive oil, vinegar, maple syrup, curry powder, and lime juice. Mix together until combined. Turn off heat and stir in the fennel, pepper, celery, and quinoa.

3. To serve, spoon quinoa chicken mixture on Boston lettuce leaves and wrap up.

Note from the Kitchen:

This recipe is perfect for a light meal (4 to 5 lettuce leaf wraps) or as a healthy appetizer.

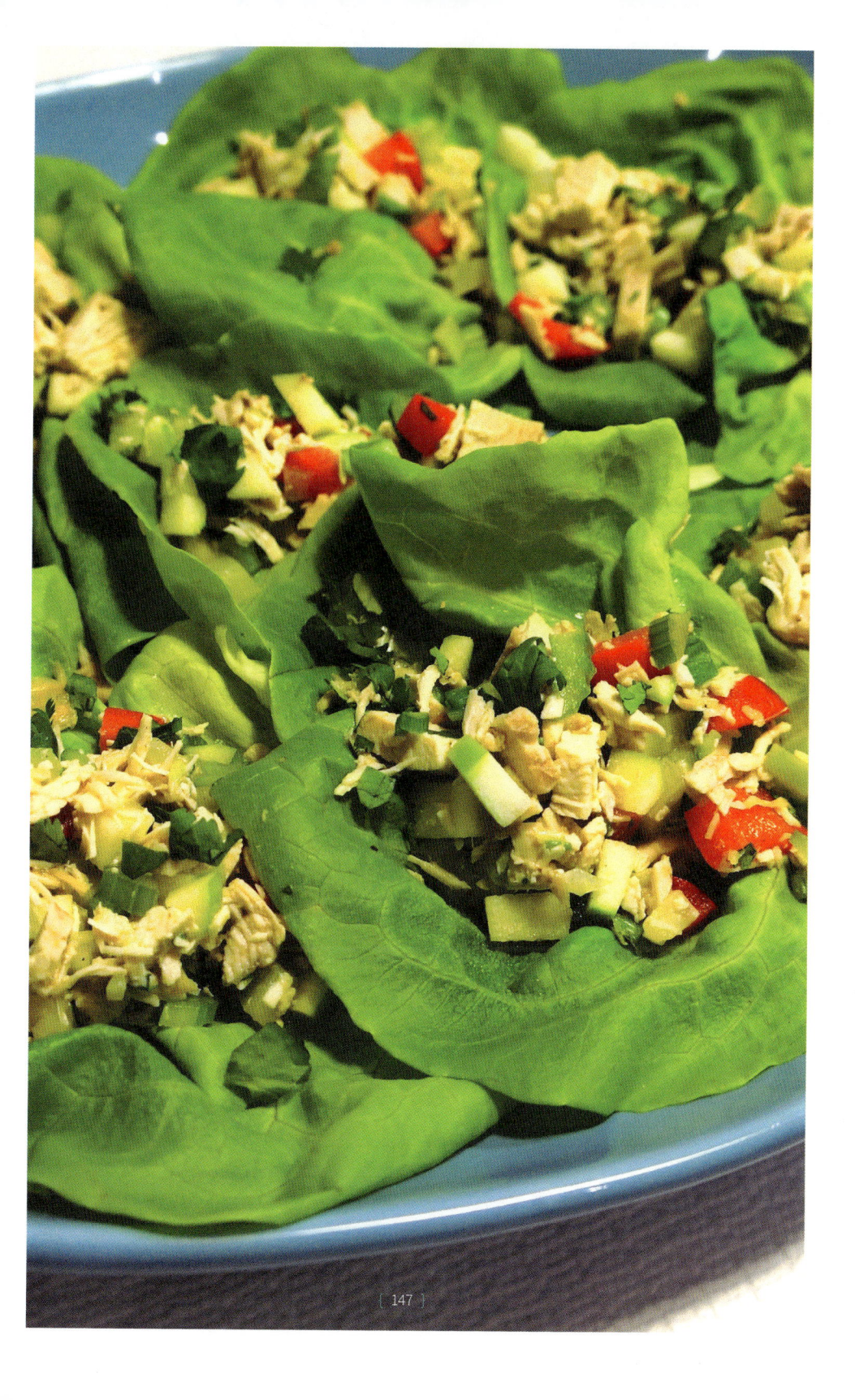

Pineapple Chicken Salad Bowl with Rice Noodles

Makes 4 servings

Prep time: 10 minutes | Cook time: 20 minutes

INGREDIENTS

1 lb boneless chicken breasts

2 tbsp tamari (gluten free)

2 tbsp sesame oil

½ pack (½ lb) rice vermicelli noodles

1 cup diced pineapple (about 3 rings)

6 cups torn pieces of leafy lettuce

1 cup cucumber slices

¼ cup peanuts

Fresh cilantro

For the dressing

1 tbsp tamari (gluten free)

1 ½ tbsp sesame oil

1 tbsp rice vinegar

Juice of 1 lime

½ tbsp maple syrup

1 green onion, diced (green part only)

INSTRUCTIONS

1. Preheat the oven to 425°F.

2. Slice the chicken breast into strips and place in a large bowl. Add tamari and sesame oil to bowl and toss to coat. Transfer to a lined baking sheet and roast for 15 to 20 minutes, until no longer pink inside. Alternatively, chicken can be grilled or pan-fried.

3. Meanwhile, bring a medium pot of water to a boil. Add the rice vermicelli and cook for 2 to 4 minutes, or according to package directions. Drain, rinse, and toss in a little sesame oil to prevent sticking. Spread noodles out on a large plate or tray to allow cooling.

4. In a small bowl whisk together the dressing ingredients and set aside until ready to use.

5. Heat a griddle pan or using your BBQ, grill pineapple slices 2 to 3 minutes per side, until grill lines are made. Flip and cook the other side. Dice into bite-size chunks and set aside. Once chicken is done cooking, remove from oven and dice.

6. Create salad bowl by layering greens, noodles, chicken, pineapple, and cucumber in a bowl. Top with peanuts, fresh cilantro, and dressing.

Note from the Kitchen:

This recipe has been built to use up leftovers from the recipe Sesame Chicken Lettuce Tacos with Rice Noodles by making a double batch of chicken and noodles in that recipe and freezing. This recipe shows you how to make the meal from scratch if you do not have the leftovers to work with.

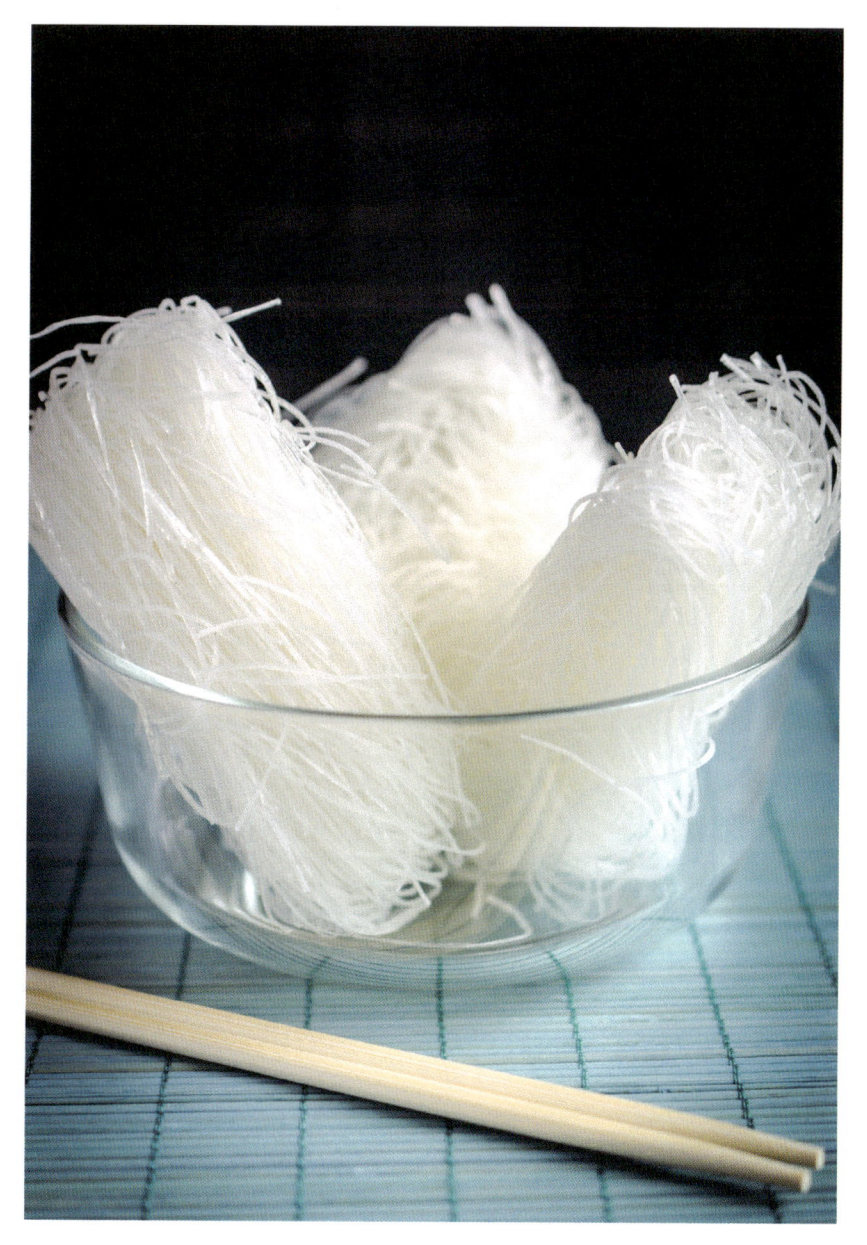

Roasted Chicken Breast

Makes 4 servings

Prep time: 5 minutes | Cook time: 35 to 45 minutes

INGREDIENTS

4 small bone-in, skin-on chicken breasts (about 1 ½ lbs OR can use slightly larger and serve half portions)

Olive oil

Salt and pepper to taste

Lemon wedges, to serve

INSTRUCTIONS

1. Preheat the oven to 425°F.
2. Place chicken breasts, skin side up, on a lined baking sheet. Drizzle with a little olive oil and rub into skin. Sprinkle with salt and pepper. Roast for 35 to 45 minutes, until cooked through and internal temperature reaches 165°F.
3. Rest for 5 to 10 minutes before serving with lemon wedges.

Note from the Kitchen:

This roasted chicken recipe is perfect with the Spring Pea Risotto and can also be served with ½ to 1 cup roasted potatoes, rice, quinoa, or other acceptable starch and 1 to 2 cups roasted vegetables or salad per person as a balanced meal.

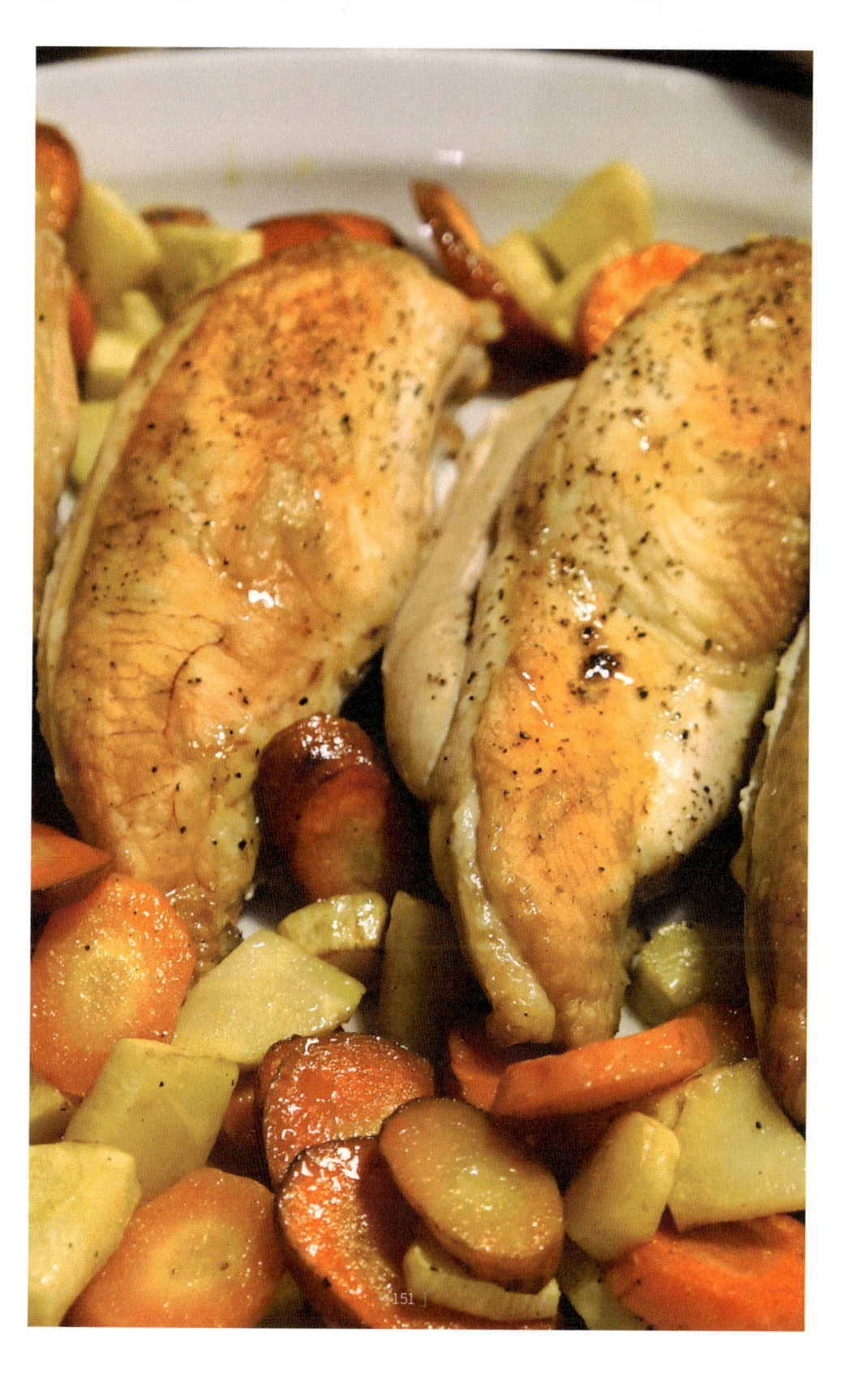

Grilled Flank Steak

Makes 4 servings

Prep time: 1 to 4 hours | Cook time: 10 minutes

INGREDIENTS

500 g flank steak of top sirloin, preferrably grass-fed

3 tbsp tamari (gluten free)

2 tbsp white wine vinegar

2 tbsp white or brown sugar

2 tbsp sesame oil

1 tsp dried oregano

1 tsp chili flakes

½ tsp paprika

½ tsp freshly ground pepper

INSTRUCTIONS

1. Whisk together all ingredients. Pour in a large freezer bag.

2. Add steak to bag, remove some of the air, and close. Place in the fridge for 1 to 4 hours, or overnight to marinade.

3. Prior to cooking remove meat from fridge and sit on the counter to allow the meat to come to room temperature (about 10 to 20 minutes). During this time preheat your grill or BBQ on medium high.

4. Place the meat directly over the flame, close the lid and turn down heat to medium-low. Cook 5 to 8 minutes on this side depending on the thickness of the meat and desired cook (medium rare vs. medium well). Lift the lid, flip the steak onto the other side and continue cooking until desired doneness is acheived.

5. Serve a starch and vegetables.

Note about Digestion:

For some, red meat can be a challenge to digest. Be aware of your body and mindful of your symptoms. Limit servings of meat to 2 to 4 oz per meal.

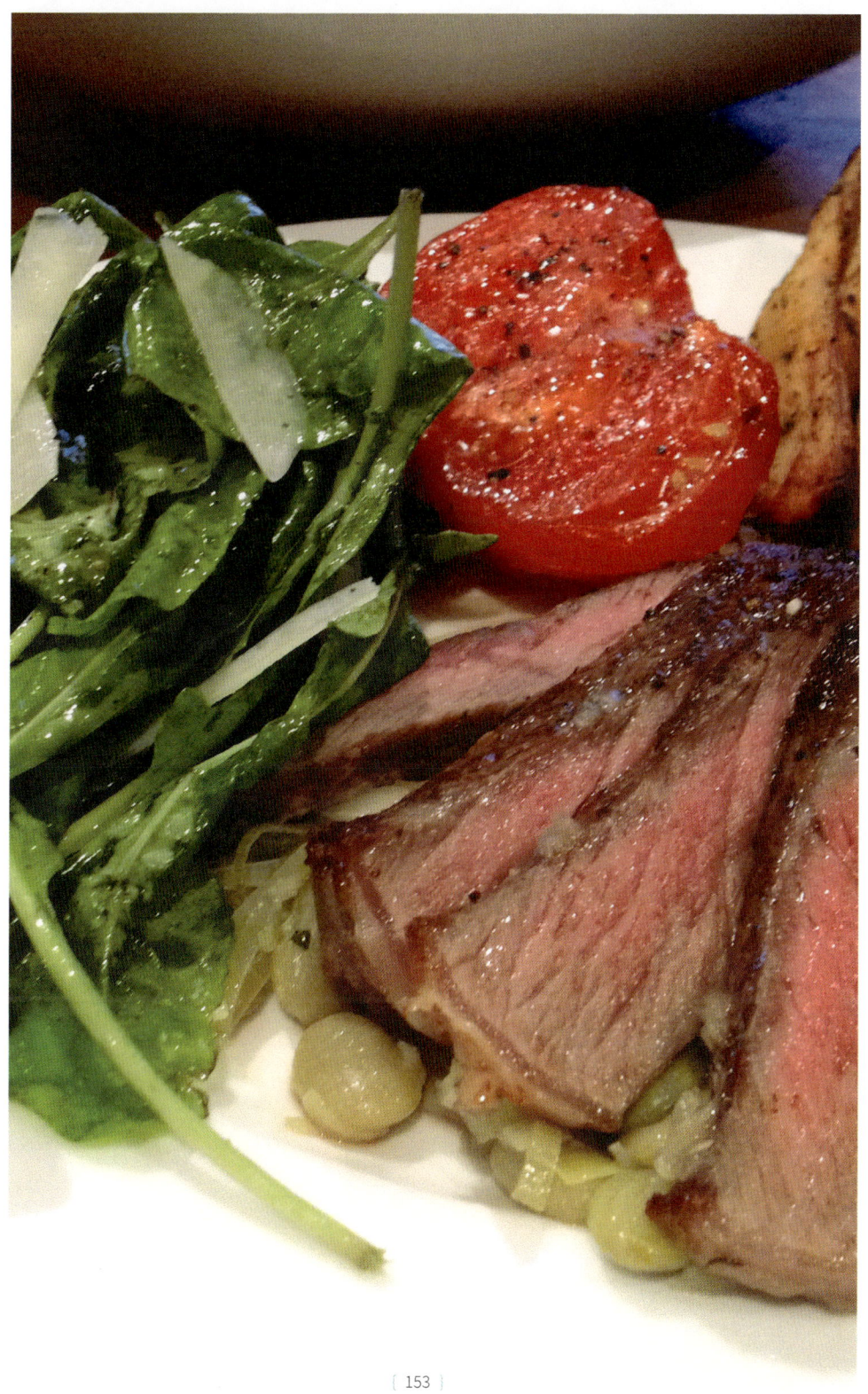

Chicken Cotoletta with Roasted Carrots and Green Beans

Makes 4 servings

Prep time: 15 minutes | Cook time: 40 minutes

INGREDIENTS

4 large (about 4 cups) carrots, sliced

1 tbsp olive oil

Salt and pepper

2 tsp maple syrup

500g boneless, skinless chicken breast (at least 2 breasts)

⅛ tsp dried cayenne, *if you like it spicy

½ cup rice flour

2 eggs, beaten

1 cup breadcrumbs (gluten free)

1 to 2 tbsp olive oil

4 cups green beans

Juice from ½–1 lemon

INSTRUCTIONS

1. Wash and slice carrots into rounds. Toss with olive oil, salt, and pepper, place in casserole dish and cover with tin foil. Cook for 20 minutes in a preheated oven at 425°F. Remove foil and continue cooking another 15 to 20 minutes until desired tenderness is reached. Toss with a little maple syrup.

2. Bring a medium pot of water to a boil.

3. Slice chicken breast horizontally through the middle to create two large, wide pieces. Flatten with a meat mallet until ½ inch thick. Season with salt and pepper (and cayenne pepper as desired). Then toss with flour, gently shake off excess. Coat with egg then place in breadcrumbs and press in firmly. Shake off excess and continue with all pieces of chicken.

4. Add olive oil to a large non-stick pan. Add chicken but be careful not to overcrowd the pan. Cook on medium heat for 3 minutes until browned, flip and finish cooking the other side.

5. Trim green beans and place in boiling water for two minutes until bright green and tender crisp. Remove and season.

6. Serve chicken with a squeeze of lemon and vegetables.

Note about Digestion:

If using cayenne, note that spicy foods can cause digestive upset for some individuals. Be aware of your body and symptoms to figure out is this is something you should avoid.

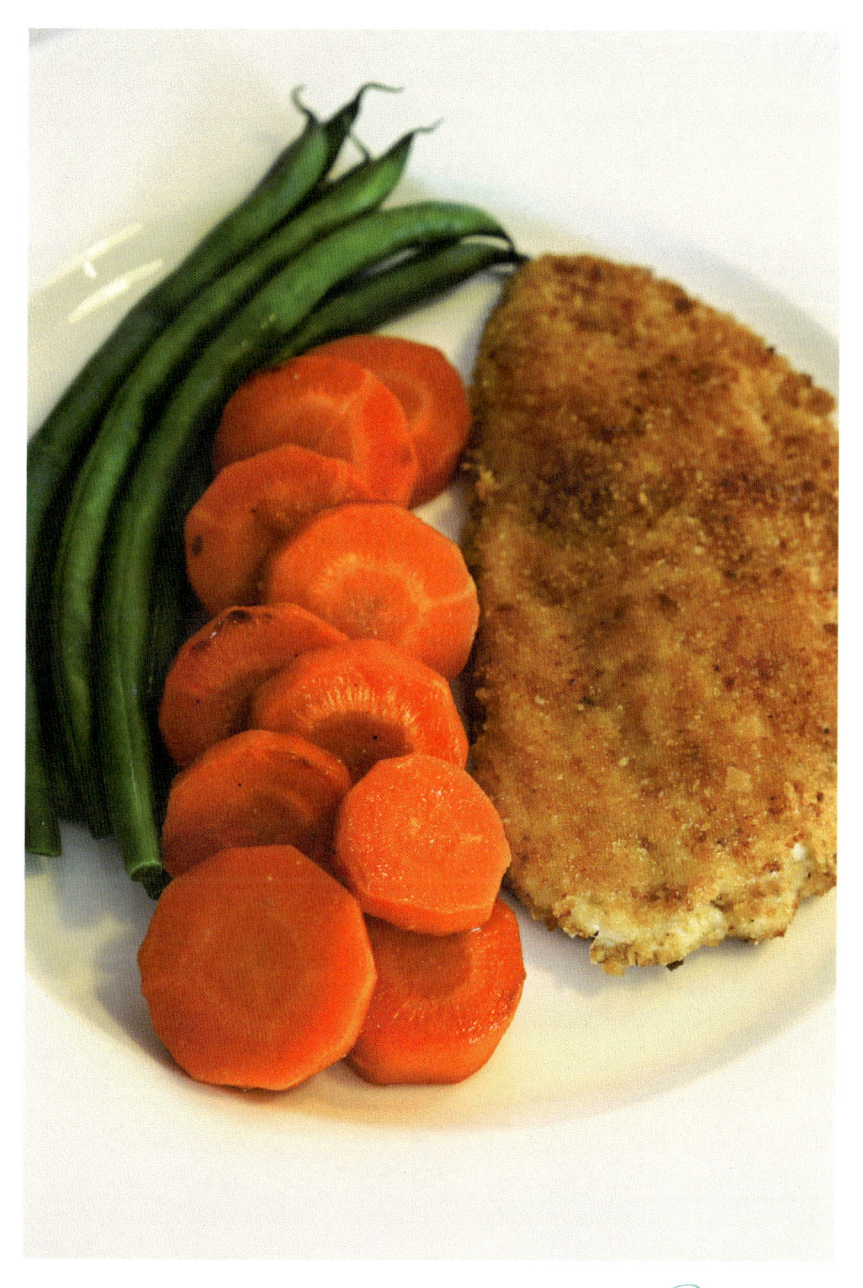

Pan-Fried Chicken Pasta with Fresh Tomato Sauce

Makes 4 servings

Prep time: 15 minutes | Cook time: 15 minutes

INGREDIENTS

1 lb boneless, skinless chicken breast

Salt and pepper to taste

2 tsp olive oil

½ lb dry pasta (gluten free), like penne, spaghetti, or fettucini

For the sauce

2 tbsp olive oil

1 cup fennel, diced

2 medium red peppers, diced

4 large (about 4 cups) tomatoes, diced

½ cup red wine

3 cups fresh spinach or other greens like kale, collards, or chard, diced

Handful of fresh basil

INSTRUCTIONS

1. Place a large pot filled with water on the stove and bring to a boil.
2. Slice chicken breasts side-to-side to create two large, wide pieces. Flatten with a meat mallet until ½ cm thick and season with salt and pepper.
3. Add 2 tsp olive oil to a large metal skillet on medium heat. Add the flattened chicken two pieces at a time (do not overcrowd the pan) and cook until it browns and easily releases from the skillet, about 2 to 4 minutes. Flip and continue cooking until no longer pink inside and nicely browned, about 2 to 3 minutes more. Remove from skillet and set aside.
4. Meanwhile, cook the pasta in the boiling water according to package directions or until al dente.

5. Make the sauce by adding the olive oil and fennel to the same hot skillet used for the chicken and cook 2 to 3 minutes. Add peppers and cook 2 minutes more. Add tomatoes and red wine, scraping little brown bits of from the bottom of the skillet. Let cook 2 to 3 minutes until wine has reduced somewhat and mixture is thick.

6. Drain the pasta and add to the skillet with the vegetables. Turn off the heat and stir in the spinach and fresh basil. Serve immediately.

Note from the Kitchen:

Serve with chicken on the side OR dice the chicken and mix with the vegetables and pasta.

Note about Digestion:

This pasta is also delicious with diced mushrooms, any kind. Mushrooms are high in the FODMAP polyol. If this is not a trigger food for you, consider adding 1 to 2 cups to the sauce.

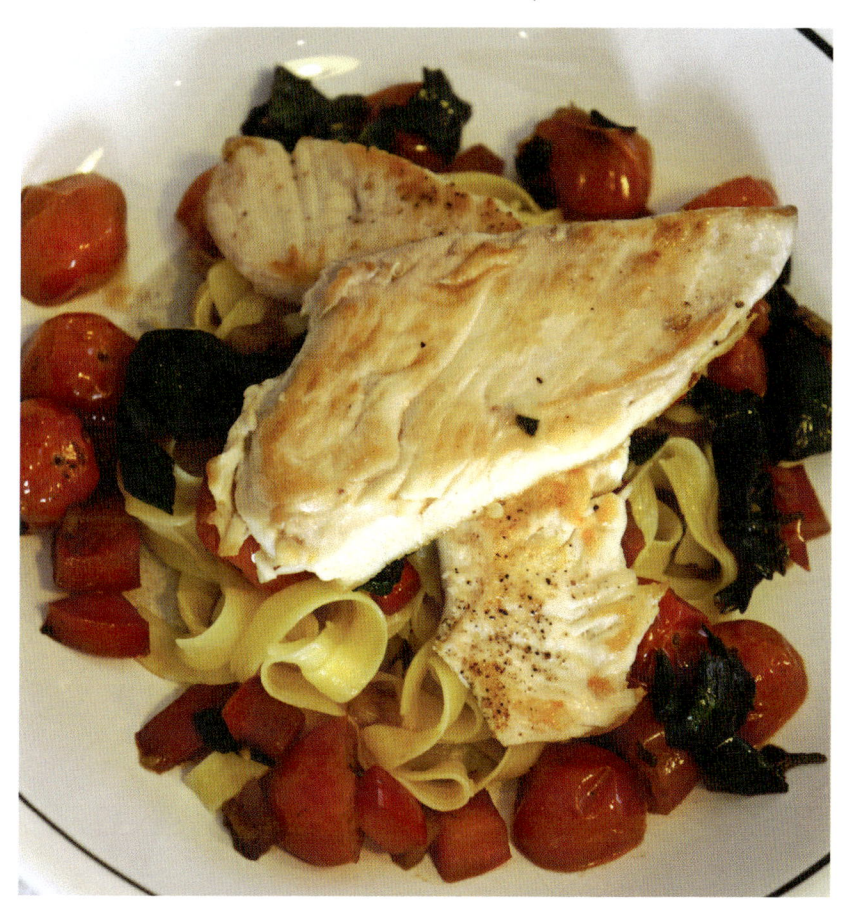

Classic Chicken Corn Fajitas

Makes 4 servings

Prep time: 10 minutes
Cook time: 30 minutes (10 minutes if using cooked chicken)

INGREDIENTS

1 lb boneless, skinless chicken breast

1 tbsp olive oil

2 tbsp white wine

8 small corn tortillas

3 large (about 3 cups) tomatoes, chopped

6 cups Boston lettuce or baby spinach, roughly shredded

1 cup microgreens or sprouts

½ avocado, diced into small pieces

Handful of fresh cilantro, chopped

2 limes

For the sauce

1 tbsp tamari (gluten free)

1 tbsp sesame oil

½ tbsp maple syrup

Hot sauce or cayenne, if tolerated

INSTRUCTIONS

1. Warm a metal skillet on medium heat. Pat off chicken with paper towel to dry and cut into ½ inch pieces. Place olive oil in the skillet and add chicken. Allow the chicken to stick to pan and create browning, about 3 to 5 minutes. Turn over and brown on the other side when chicken releases from the pan. Once chicken is cooked through (total time of 5 to 8 minutes), add wine to deglaze the pan. Alternatively cook whole chicken breasts in a preheated oven at 425°F for 25 to 30 minutes and chop once cooled slightly.

2. Warm the tortillas in microwave or oven at 225°F until soft. If warming in the oven, cover with tin foil to prevent the tortillas from hardening.

3. Place cooked chicken in each tortilla, add toppings and sauce. Fold both sides in and enjoy! Use extra vegetable ingredients to make a side salad. Top with a little lime juice, olive oil, and salt and pepper.

Note from the Kitchen:

These fajitas can also be served with ground pork, beef, chicken, turkey, pan-fried fish, or crumbled tempeh! Enjoy with your favourite toppings or stir-fry some peppers, eggplant, and spinach as a topping instead of raw vegetables.

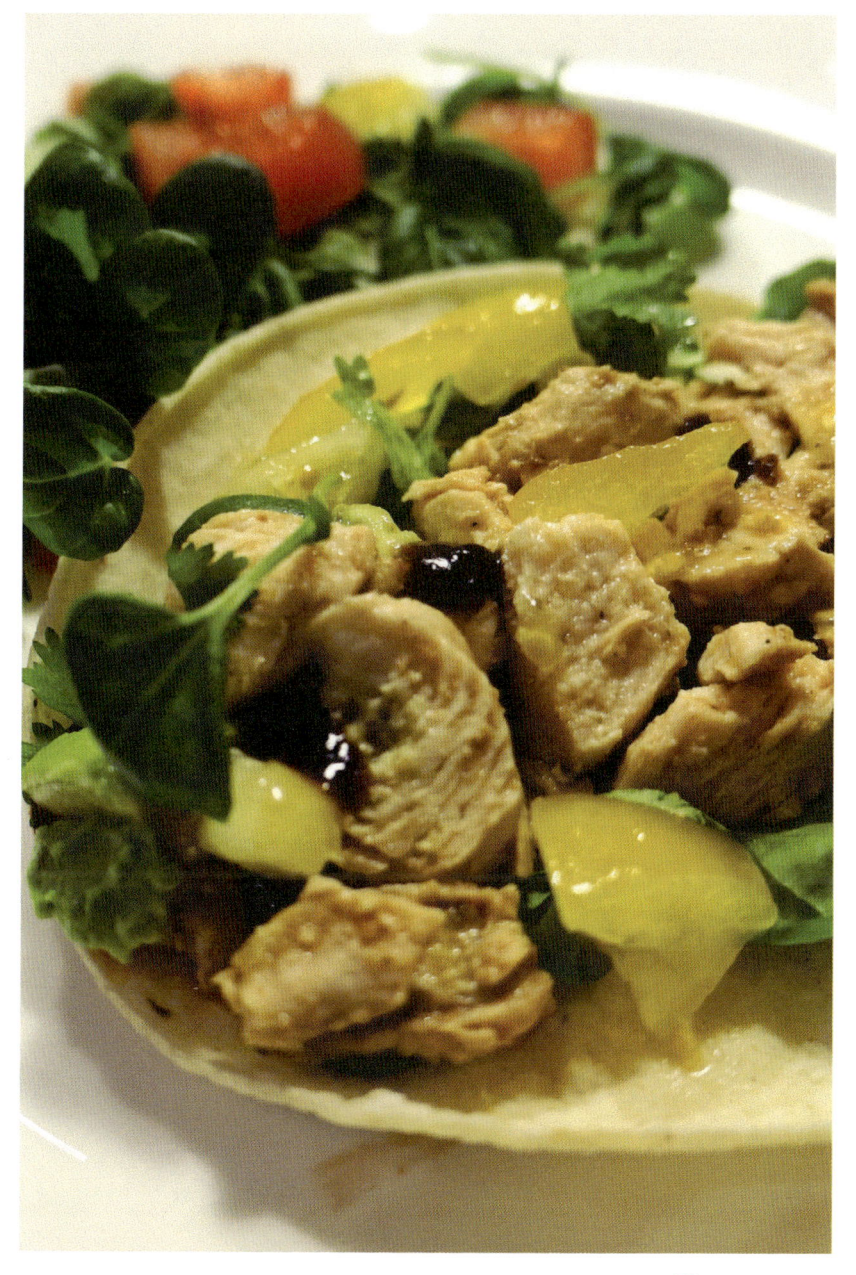

Beef and Vegetable Burritos

Makes 4 servings

Prep time: 15 minutes | Cook time: 15 minutes

INGREDIENTS

1 lb extra lean ground beef

½ cup red wine

2 tsp olive oil

1 stalk celery, diced

½ cup fennel, diced

½ cup green beans, diced into small pieces

1 large (about 1 cup) red pepper, diced

½ tsp EACH dried coriander, oregano, chili powder

½ tsp EACH dried cumin, smoked paprika

Pinch of salt, pepper, cayenne

4 large gluten-free tortillas

½ cup old cheddar cheese, grated *optional

Optional toppings:

Diced avocado, tomato, fresh lime, and/or fresh cilantro

Tofutti (vegan brand) sour cream to serve

INSTRUCTIONS

1. Preheat the oven to 400°F.
2. Heat a large metal skillet on medium-high heat. Flatten and dry surface of ground beef with a paper towel. Place into hot pan. Allow to brown for 2 to 4 minutes, before flipping over. Cook beef until browned and cooked through (about 5 minutes). Deglaze pan with red wine, scraping up all brown bits from pan and remove.
3. Add olive oil, celery and fennel to hot pan. Sauté 3 to 4 minutes. Add green beans and red pepper. Cook 3 minutes more. Add herbs, spices, and meat to the vegetables and mix through.
4. Meanwhile, warm 4 large gluten-free tortillas (i.e. made with teff, rice, or corn flour) in the microwave or wrapped in tinfoil in the oven for a few minutes.
5. Once beef mixture is done, place a small amount of cheese (*if using) in the center of the wrap and ¼ of the beef/vegetable mixture on top. Roll and place on a cookie sheet seam-side down. Place in oven and cook 5 to 7 minutes until crispy.
6. Serve with diced avocado, tomato, cilantro, lime, and Tofutti (vegan) sour cream if desired.

Note about Digestion:

For some individuals, spices and red meat can be difficult to digest. You may want to alter this recipe to use less spice if this is a concern—try ¼ tsp of each ingredient instead of ½ tsp. If red meat causes digestive distress, than opt for ground chicken, turkey, or crumbled tempeh in this recipe instead of beef.

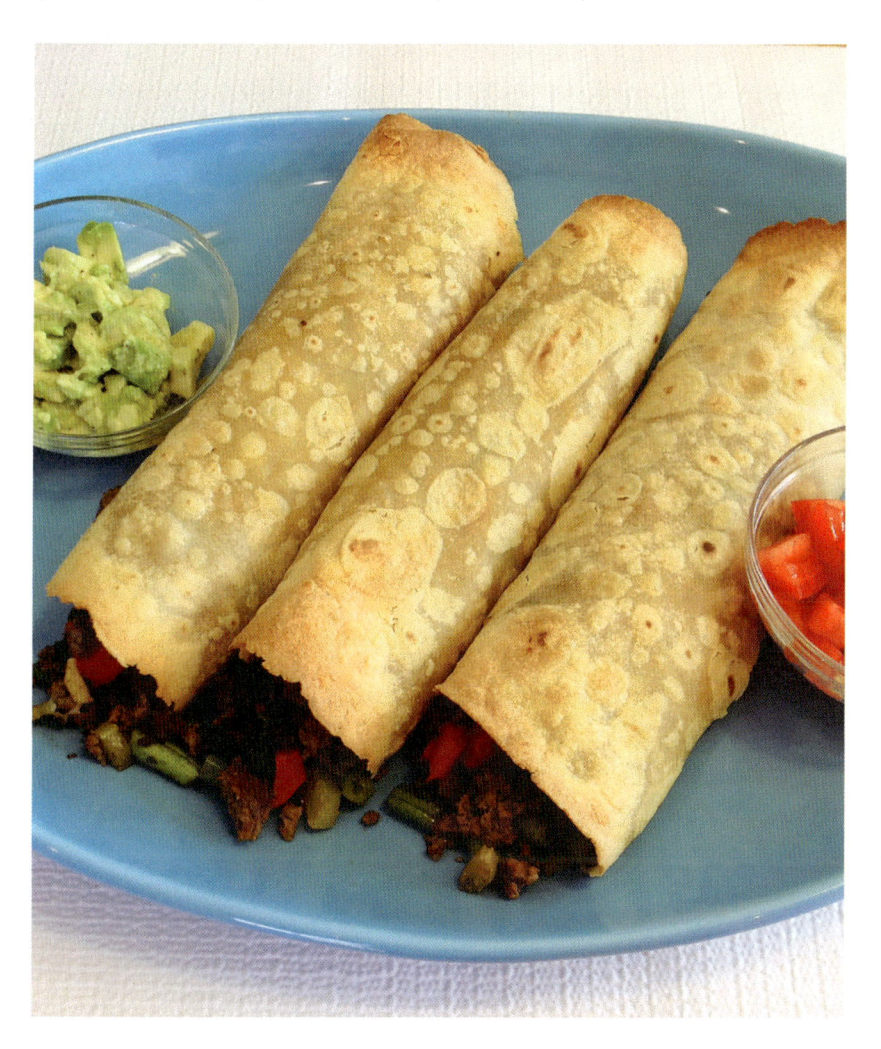

Chili Chicken Stuffed Peppers

Makes 4 servings

Prep time: 15 minutes | Cook time: 45 minutes

INGREDIENTS

4 large red, yellow, or orange bell peppers

Olive oil to rub in peppers

1 cup long grain or wild rice mix like Lundberg brand (4 cups cooked)

1 lb ground chicken

¼ cup white wine (or water)

1 tbsp olive oil

1 cup fennel, diced

1 cup kale, spinach, or collards, shredded

¼ tsp chili flakes

1 tsp EACH dried parsley, thyme, sage

½ tsp chili powder

Freshly ground pepper

4 tomatoes, diced

¼ cup OLD cheddar cheese, shredded *optional

INSTRUCTIONS

1. Preheat oven to 425°F.

2. Cut peppers in half from stem to bottom and remove seeds. Rub in olive oil and place on a baking sheet. Roast in oven for 20 minutes turning halfway through cooking time.

3. Meanwhile, prepare rice as per packet instructions. Generally, 1 cup white rice to 1¼ cups water OR 1 cup long grain or brown rice to 1 ½ to 2 cups water.

4. Heat a large, metal, deep sauté pan on medium high heat. Add chicken and allow sticking to the pan to create browning. Stir after a couple minutes when meat releases from pan. Cook until browned. Add ¼ cup wine or water to deglaze the pan, scraping all the little brown bits up. Remove from pan. Place pan back on heat.

5. Add 1 tbsp olive oil and fennel to hot sauté pan. Cook for 5 minutes. Add kale or other greens and chili flakes, parsley, thyme, sage, chili powder, and pepper. Cook for 5 minutes more. Add tomatoes and cook for 2 minutes more. Add the meat back to the pan and cooked rice to the mix, stir to combine.

6. Remove peppers from oven once cooked but still firm. Pack chicken and rice mixture evenly into each pepper. Top with cheese if using. Broil in oven until cheese is melted—approximately 2 minutes.

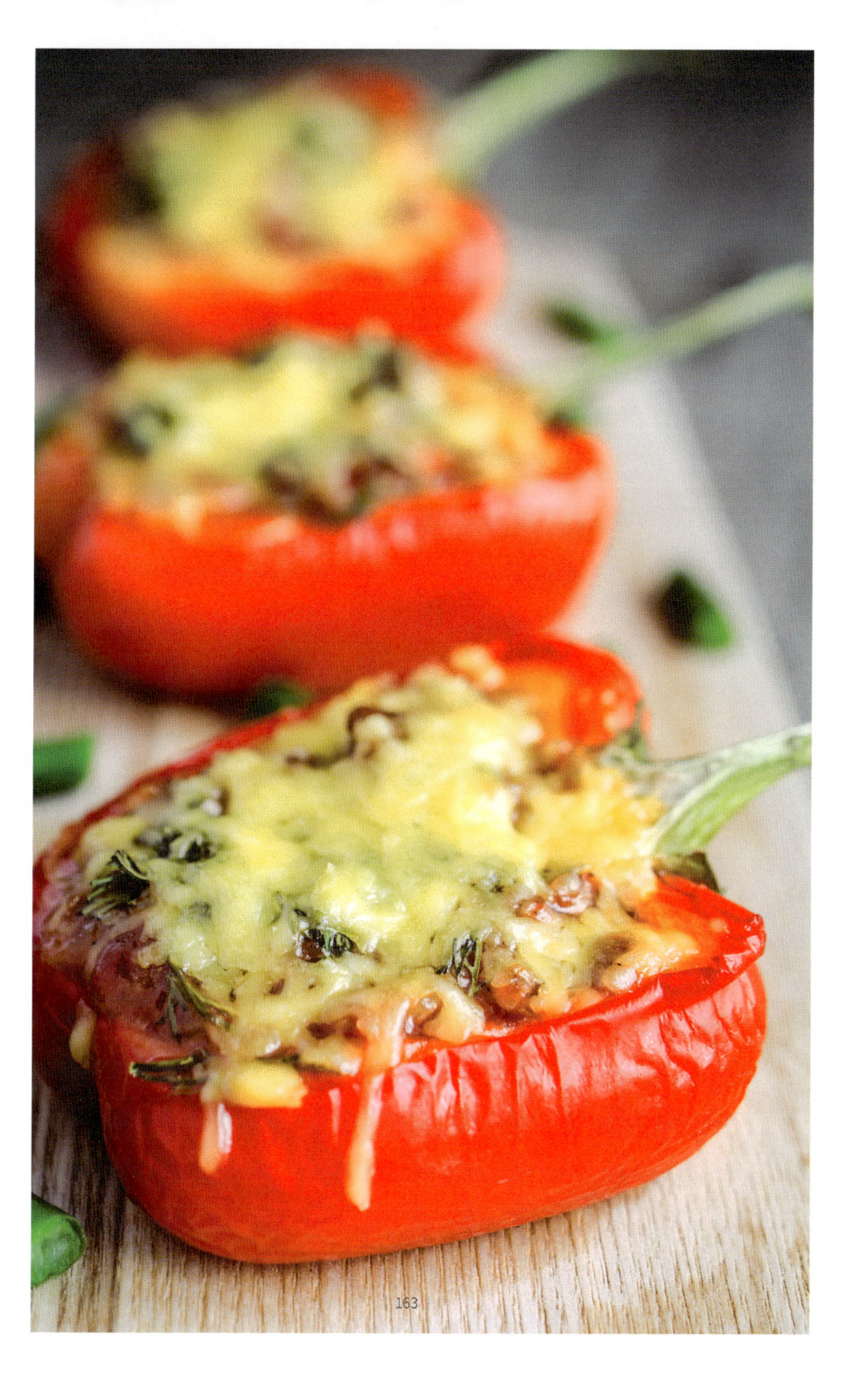

Simple Beef Burgers

Makes 4 burgers

Prep time: 5 minutes (PLUS chill time of at least one hour)
Cook time: 10 to 15 minutes

INGREDIENTS

500 g ground beef chuck, preferably grass-fed and local

1 tbsp red wine

1 tsp tamari (gluten free)

1 tsp balsamic vinegar

1 tsp red pepper flakes or Epicure Selections 5 pepper blend

Freshly ground pepper (about ¼ tsp)

4 gluten free buns

INSTRUCTIONS

1. In a large bowl combine beef, wine, tamari, vinegar, pepper flakes, and ground pepper mixing gently. Be careful not to over mix, which will affect the texture of the burger.

2. Divide the meat mixture evenly into 4 portions. (You can use a kitchen scale to ensure equal weight. Press the meat portions into patties about ½ inch thick, making a small dip in the middle to allow for expansion. Preferably, allow 1 hour for refrigeration before cooking, however the burgers can be cooked straight away as well.

3. Heat a grill or barbecue to high. As soon as you add the patties, turn heat to medium and close lid. Check burgers after 4 to 6 minutes and flip just once when they release from the grill. Do not poke or squish burgers. Use a thermometer to check for internal temperature of 160°C.

4. Transfer to a clean plate, allow resting for 5 minutes, and serve on a gluten-free bun with simple condiments such as lettuce, tomato, mustard, mayonnaise, and/or pickles and a salad or grilled vegetables for a balanced meal.

Note from the Kitchen:

Alternatively, you can grill the burgers on an iron grill pan on the stove top on medium-high heat. Place the burgers on the pan and cook for 2 to 3 minutes per side. Rotate 90 degrees to make grill lines. Cook 1 to 2 minutes more and flip. Place in a preheated oven at 375°F for 4 to 7 minutes until cooked through.

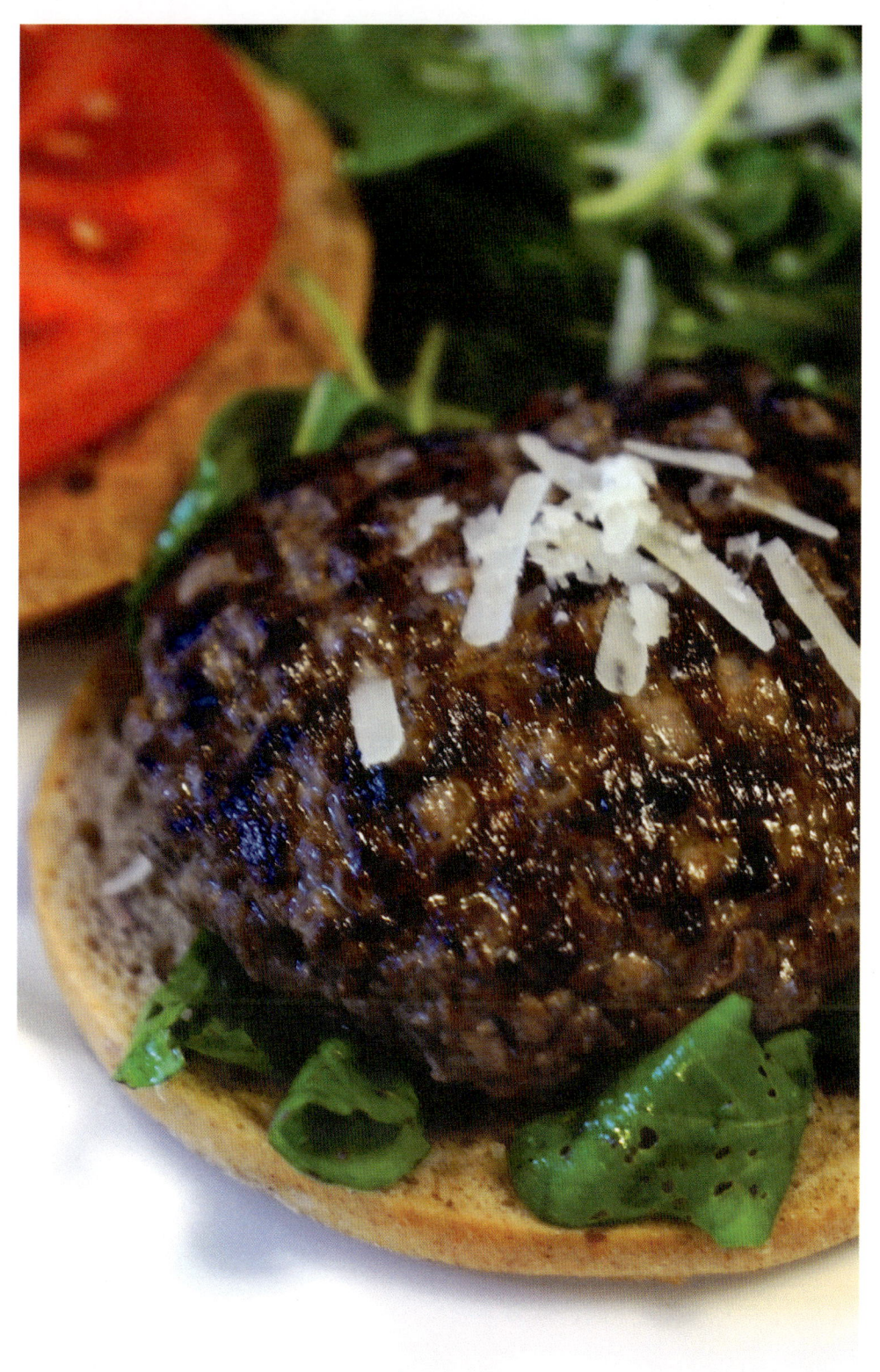

The Best Turkey Burgers

Makes 8 servings

Prep time: 15 minutes | Cook time: 45 minutes

INGREDIENTS

- 2 tsp garlic infused olive oil
- 2 tbsp fennel, minced
- 2 tbsp yellow bell pepper, minced
- 1 tsp dried basil
- 1 tsp dried parsley
- 1 tbsp lemon juice (½ a lemon)
- 1 tbsp fresh cilantro, minced
- 1 tsp Dijon mustard
- Salt and pepper
- 2 lbs ground turkey
- 1 egg, lightly beaten
- ½ cup cornmeal
- 8 gluten free buns

INSTRUCTIONS

1. Place a small frying pan on medium heat. Add garlic infused oil, fennel, and pepper. Sauté for 3 to 5 minutes until the vegetables begin to soften. Add to a large bowl and add rest of ingredients. Gently mix until all ingredients are combined.
2. Form 8 equal size patties and chill in freezer for at least one hour, 3 to 4 hours is preferable.
3. In an iron skillet on the stove top or using a BBQ or grill, cook on medium heat until cooked through. If cooking on the stove top, you may want to finish the burgers in the oven at 375°F for 10 to 12 minutes, once browned on the outside. If using a BBQ or grill, the burgers will take 15 to 20 minutes. The burgers are done once a meat thermometer reads an internal temperature of 165°F. Flip just once during cooking. Do not push down on burgers to allow cooking without squishing out liquid.
4. Enjoy with a fresh gluten-free bun and leafy salad.

Note from the Kitchen:

This recipe makes 8 burgers, so you can freeze the extras. If you're making them anyways, might as well make a double batch!

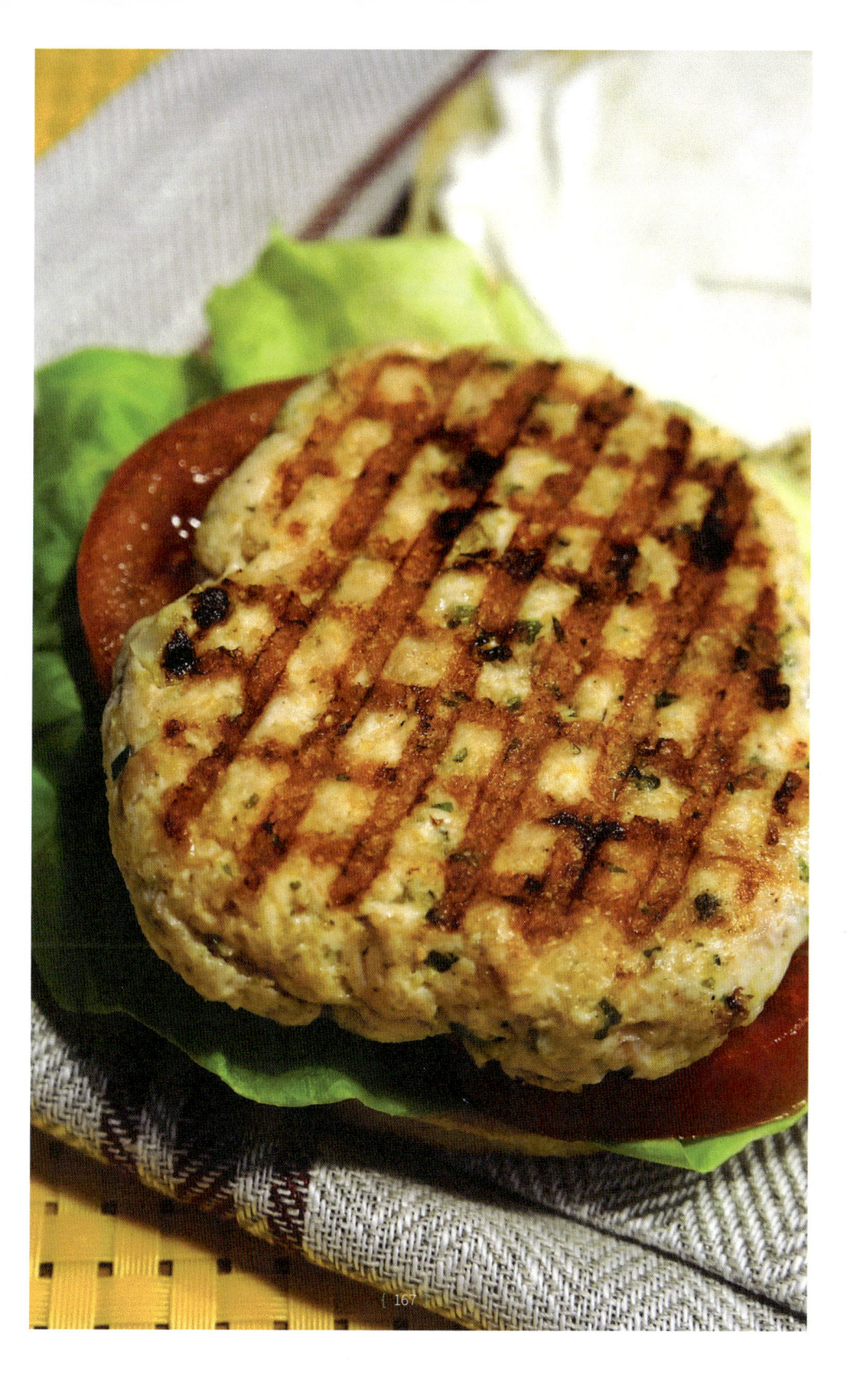

Chapter Three

The IBS MASTER PLAN

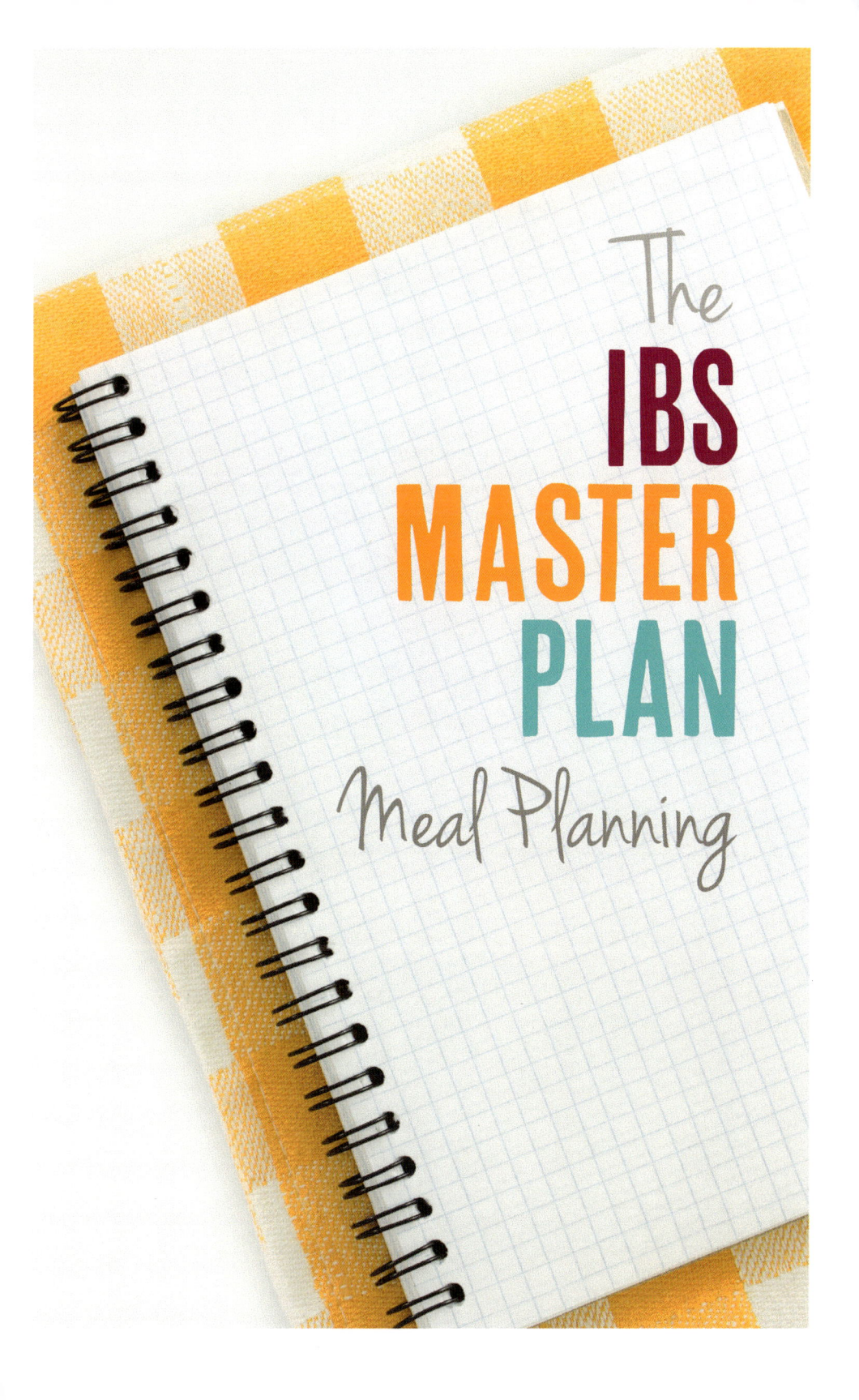

Meal Planning

Meal Plan Week One

	MONDAY	TUESDAY	WEDNESDAY
BREAKFAST	Amazing Oatmeal Recipe of Choice	Tasty Toast Balanced Breakfast of Choice	Sensational Smoothie Recipe of Choice
LUNCH	**Make-ahead** Roasted Red Pepper Pasta Salad	**Leftover** Roasted Red Pepper Pasta Salad	BLT sandwich using **leftover tempeh bacon** and a side of vegetables/salad
Notes	Make double for Tuesday lunch.		
SUPPER	Grilled Pickerel with Spanish Quinoa Side Salad	Spinach Salad Bowls with Tempeh Bacon	Sesame Chicken Lettuce Tacos with Rice Noodles
Notes	Make 2 cups (cooked) extra quinoa for Thursday dinner.	Make double recipe of tempeh bacon (for tomorrow's lunch) & double portion of sweet potato (for Friday lunch).	Make double recipe for Thursday lunch. Also make 1 lb extra chicken & ½ pack extra rice noodles to freeze for next Wednesday dinner.

THURSDAY	FRIDAY	SATURDAY	SUNDAY
Amazing Oatmeal Recipe of Choice	Tasty Toast Balanced Breakfast of Choice	Amazing Oatmeal Recipe of Choice	Fabulous French Toast or Pancake Recipe of Choice
Leftover Sesame Chicken Lettuce Tacos with Rice Noodles	Leafy salad using **leftover** sweet potato **(Tues)** and **leftover** crunchy tofu **(Thurs)**	Roasted Red Pepper Tuna Quinoa Cakes with vegetable salad	Leafy Italian Salad with Quinoa
		Make double recipe of Tuna Cakes & freeze.	Make 2 cups (cooked) extra quinoa for Thursday dinner.
Crunchy Cornmeal-Crusted Tofu in Collard Wraps with Quinoa	Roasted Chicken Breast and Spring Pea Risotto	Simple Beef Burgers with leafy salad	Grilled sausages (GF) or fish with Grilled Vegetables and Potatoes
Use leftover quinoa from Monday. Make a double batch of crunchy tofu for Friday lunch. Make double recipe of chipotle mayo.	Make double roasted chicken for Thursday dinner. Cool, dice, & freeze.	Double recipe and freeze half for another meal.	Make double recipe for Monday lunch.

Grocery List Week One

Notes

Groceries are based on meals for four people. There is enough oatmeal for 3 breakfasts, 2 slices of toast for 3 breakfasts and 1 lunch. Ingredients are not included for salads for Wednesday, Friday, and Saturday lunch OR for Monday and Saturday supper. Make sure to add ingredients to your shopping list for these extra items.

Produce	Quantity
*Fruit for breakfast smoothies and snacks	
*Extra produce for five salads	
Red, Yellow, or Orange Bell Pepper	9
Yellow Zucchini	6
Fennel Bulb	3
Kale	8 cups
Cherry Tomatoes	6 cups
Lemon	7
Sweet Potato	4 medium (about 4 cups)
Baby Spinach	12 cups
Carrot	4 large
Cucumber	1
Tomato	1 large
Boston Lettuce	3 heads
Green Onion	1 bunch
Lime	3
Collard Leaves	1 bunch (about 8 leaves)
Fresh (or Frozen) Peas	1 cup
Sprouts or Micro-greens	1 cup
Fresh Basil	1 bunch
Fresh Cilantro	1 bunch
Small New or Red Potatoes	8 cups

Grains	Quantity
Oatmeal	About 6 cups (dry)
Gluten Free Bread	32 slices (≈8 slices/ person)
Gluten Free Burger Buns	4
Gluten Free Penne	6 cups
Quinoa	7 cups
Rice Vermicelli Noodles	1 pack
Cornmeal	1 cup
Arborio Rice	1 cup
Gluten Free Bread Crumbs	1 cup

Meat & Alternatives	Quantity
Fresh Pickerel (buy 1-2 days before cooking)	1 ½ lbs
Tempeh	2 blocks (about 250 g each)
Chicken Breast, boneless, skinless	3 lbs
Chicken Breast, bone-in, skin-on	3 lbs
Firm Tofu, preferably organic	2 blocks (450 g each)
Canned Tuna, flaked (in water)	4 cans
Eggs, large	2 (plus more for breakfast)
Ground Beef Chuck	1 kg
Chickpeas	2 cans
Sausage (ask for GF and least garlic/onions)	8 (about 2 ½ lbs)
Sesame Seeds	¼ cup
Pine Nuts	1 ¼ cup
*Nuts and seeds for snacks	
Boston Lettuce	3 heads

Dairy	Quantity
Parmesan or Grana Padano cheese	5 to 6 oz
Mayonnaise (or Veganaise)	About 1 cup
Butter or Earth Balance Margarine	As needed

Other	Quantity
Jar of Roasted Red Peppers	Need 4 peppers in total
Chipotle Pepper in Adobo Sauce	1 Pepper
Vegetable or Chicken Stock	1 L
White Wine	½ cup
Red Wine	⅛ cup
Walnut oil	½ tbsp

*Additional items that have not been calculated into the shopping list.
Calculate how many of each you will need for your family depending on your likes, dislikes, meals, and snacks.

Meal Plan Week Two

	MONDAY	TUESDAY	WEDNESDAY
BREAKFAST	Amazing Oatmeal Recipe of Choice	Tasty Toast Balanced Breakfast of Choice	Sensational Smoothie Recipe of Choice
LUNCH	Leftover Sausage, vegetables, and potatoes	Leftover Tempeh taco wraps (leftover tempeh on corn tortillas with salad	Make ahead Roasted Vegetable Lentil Salad
Notes			Make double for Thursday lunch.
SUPPER	Tempeh Taco Salad	Breaded Cod with Rice Pilaf and grilled vegetables OR salad	Rice noodle bowls with chicken and veggies
Notes	*Make 2 cups (cooked) extra quinoa for Thursday dinner.*	*Take out chicken and noodles to defrost.*	*Use leftover chicken & noodle from last Wednesday.* *Take out chicken to defrost.*

THURSDAY	FRIDAY	SATURDAY	SUNDAY
Amazing Oatmeal Recipe of Choice	Tasty Toast Balanced Breakfast of Choice	Amazing Oatmeal Recipe of Choice	Fabulous French Toast or Pancake Recipe of Choice
Leftover Roasted Vegetable Lentil Salad	**Leftover** Roasted Red Pepper Tuna Quinoa Cakes with vegetable salad	Egg salad sandwich with sliced vegetables	Simple Rice Paper Salad Rolls
Curry Chicken Salad Lettuce Wraps	Homemade pizza night (use Udi's or other GF pizza crust) with Protein Power Side Salad	Grilled Flank Steak with Grilled Vegetables and Potatoes	Pan-Fried Chicken Pasta with Fresh Tomato Sauce
Use leftover diced chicken from Friday dinner and leftover quinoa from Sunday lunch. Take out Tuna Cakes to defrost.			

Grocery List Week Two

Notes

Groceries are based on meals for four people. There is enough oatmeal for 3 breakfasts, 2 slices of toast for 3 breakfasts and 1 lunch. Ingredients are not included for salads/vegetables for Thursday and Friday supper or Saturday lunch as well as toppings for pizza on Friday. Make sure to add ingredients to your shopping list for these extra items.

Leftovers

If you are following these meal plans in order, you will have some leftovers saved from week one, if not, you will need the following additional items: 2 lbs cooked chicken, 2 cups cooked quinoa, and ½ pack cooked vermicelli noodles.

Produce	Quantity
*Fruit for breakfast smoothies and snacks	
*Extra produce for 3 meals	
Red, Yellow, or Orange Pepper	10
Seasonal Leafy Greens	6 cups
Fennel Bulb	2
Green Zucchini	2 medium (4 cups)
Yellow Zucchini	2 medium
Cherry Tomatoes	6 cups
Lemon	1
Avocado	1
Orange	1 large
Carrot	2 large
Cucumber	2
Radish	2
Leafy Lettuce	6 cups
Green Onion	1 bunch
Lime	2
Melon	1 medium (4 cups)
Celery	1 head (4 stalks)
Boston Lettuce	1 Head
Pineapple	3 Rings
Alfalfa Sprouts or Shredded Lettuce	1 cup
Tomato	5 large (5 cups)
Spinach, Kale, Collards, or Chard	2 cups
Fresh basil	1 bunch
Fresh cilantro	1 bunch
Small New or Red Potatoes	4 cups

Dairy	Quantity
Old Sharp Cheddar Cheese	¼ cup
Mayonnaise (or Veganaise)	As needed
Butter or Earth Balance Margarine	As needed

Meat & Alternatives	Quantity
Tempeh	2 blocks (about 250 g each)
Lentils	2 cans (3 cups)
Chicken Breasts, boneless, skinless	1 lb
Fresh Cod, boneless, skinless	500-600g
Eggs, large	1 (plus more for breakfast)
Flank Steak	1 lb
Chicken, Shrimp or Tofu (for Sunday lunch)	1 lb
Walnuts	1 cup
Peanuts	¼ cup
*Nuts & Seeds for Snacks	

Grains	Quantity
Oatmeal	About 6 cups
Gluten Free Bread	32 slices (≈8 slices/ person)
Gluten Free Nacho Chips	1 Bag
Small Corn Tortillas	8 small
Quinoa	5 Cups
Jasmine or Basmati Rice	1 Cup
White Rice Flour	⅛ Cup
Gluten Free Bread Crumbs	½ Cup
Udi's (or other GF) Pizza Crusts	1 pack
Rice Paper Sheets	12
Gluten Free Pasta	½ lb dry

Other	Quantity
Curry Powder (i.e. S&B brand)	1 tbsp
White Wine	1 cup
Red Wine	½ cup
White Sugar	
Corn Starch	

*Additional items that have not been calculated into the shopping list.
Calculate how many of each you will need for your family depending on your likes, dislikes, meals, and snacks.

Meal Plan Week Three

	MONDAY	TUESDAY	WEDNESDAY
BREAKFAST	Amazing Oatmeal Recipe of Choice	Tasty Toast Balanced Breakfast of Choice	Sensational Smoothie Recipe of Choice
LUNCH	**Make Ahead** Lemon Dill Tuna Pasta Salad	**Leftover** Roasted Chicken Breast with Grilled Vegetables and Potatoes	**Leftover** Pan-Fried Cod with Vegetable Quinoa
SUPPER	Roasted Chicken Breast with Grilled Vegetables and Potatoes	Pan-Fried Cod with Vegetable Quinoa	Classic Chicken Corn Fajitas
Notes	Make double recipe for Tuesday lunch. Also make 3 lbs extra roasted chicken for Wednesday dinner and Thursday lunch.		Use leftover chicken from Monday dinner. Double recipe for Thursday lunch.

THURSDAY	FRIDAY	SATURDAY	SUNDAY
Amazing Oatmeal Recipe of Choice	Tasty Toast Balanced Breakfast of Choice	Amazing Oatmeal Recipe of Choice	Fabulous French Toast or Pancake Recipe of Choice
Leftover Classic Chicken Corn Fajitas	**Leftover** Stupendous Superfood Minestrone	**Leftovers** Beef and Vegetable Burritos	Shrimp Burgers with Tomato Avocado Salsa and a side salad
Stupendous Superfood Minestrone	Beef and Vegetable Burritos	Smokey Tempeh and Lentil Chili with GF toast or Bob's Red Mill GF cornbread	Chili Chicken Stuffed Peppers
Make double recipe for Friday lunch.	Make double recipe for Saturday lunch.	Make double recipe for Monday lunch.	Make double recipe for Tuesday lunch.

Grocery List Week Three

Notes

*Groceries are based on meals for four people.
There is enough oatmeal for 3 breakfasts, 2 slices of toast for 3 breakfasts and 1 lunch.
Ingredients are not included for side vegetables on Monday supper or Sunday lunch.
Make sure to add ingredients to your shopping list for these extra items.*

Produce	Quantity
*Fruit for breakfast smoothies and snacks	
*Extra produce for two meals	
Lemon	5
Lime	6
Celery	1 bunch (8 stalks)
Fennel Bulb	2 large or 4 small bulbs
Kale	2 bunches (about 8 cups)
Cherry Tomatoes	4 cups
Tomato	21 large
Cucumber	1
Red, Yellow, or Orange Bell Pepper	22
Yellow Zucchini	4
Carrot	4
Eggplant	2 medium
Boston Lettuce or Baby Spinach	12 cups
Green Onion	1 bunch
Green Beans	1 cup
Avocado	3
Fresh Parsley	1 bunch
Fresh Cilantro	1 bunch
Fresh Dill	1 bunch
Sprouts or Micro-greens	2 cups
Potatoes	12 cups

Dairy	Quantity
Old Cheddar Cheese	1 ½ cups
Mayonnaise (or Veganaise)	2 tbsp
Tofutti Sour Cream	3-4 tbsp (as garnish)
Parmesan or Grana Padano	2 to 3 oz (as garnish *optional)

Meat & Alternatives	Quantity
Chicken Breast, Bone-in, Skin-on	6 lbs (about 8 to 10)
Ground Chicken	2 lbs
Ground Beef, Extra Lean	2 lbs
Bacon or pancetta	4 strips
Fresh Cod	3 lbs
Flaked Tuna (in water)	1 can
Shrimp	1.5 lbs
Eggs, large	4 (plus more for breakfast)
Lentils	1 can (2 cups)
Chickpeas	1 can (2 cups)
Tempeh	2 blocks (250 g each)
*Nuts and seeds for snacks	

Grains	Quantity
Oatmeal	About 6 cups
Gluten Free Bread	24 slices (≈6 slices/person)
Gluten Free Burger buns	4
Gluten Free Penne (or Shells)	2 cups
Gluten Free Tortillas, Large	8
Corn Tortillas, Small	16
Quinoa	4 ½ cups
Long Grain or Wild Rice Mix	2 cups
Bob's Red Mill corn bread mix	1 package

Other	Quantity
Crushed Tomatoes (Roasted)	2 cans
Red Wine	2 cup
White Wine	¾ cup

*Additional items that have not been calculated into the shopping list.
Calculate how many of each you will need for your family depending on your likes, dislikes, meals, and snacks.

Meal Plan Week Four

	MONDAY	TUESDAY	WEDNESDAY
BREAKFAST	Amazing Oatmeal Recipe of Choice	Tasty Toast Balanced Breakfast of Choice	Sensational Smoothie Recipe of Choice
LUNCH	**Leftover** Smokey Tempeh and Lentil Chili with GF toast or Bob's Red Mill GF cornbread	**Leftover** Chili Chicken Stuffed Peppers	**Leftover** Easy Lentil Quesadillas with a leafy salad
Notes			
SUPPER	Perfect Peanut Noodle Bowl	Easy Lentil Quesadillas with a leafy salad	The Best Turkey Burgers with a side salad
Notes		Make double for Wednesday lunch.	Make double for Thursday lunch. Can make this recipe ahead for a busy night.

THURSDAY	FRIDAY	SATURDAY	SUNDAY
Amazing Oatmeal Recipe of Choice	Tasty Toast Balanced Breakfast of Choice	Amazing Oatmeal Recipe of Choice	Fabulous French Toast or Pancake Recipe of Choice
Leftover The Best Turkey Burgers with a side salad	Salmon Kale Salad Sandwich with side vegetables	**Leftover** Vegetarian Vegetable Bolognese	Egg salad sandwich with sliced tomato
	Use leftover salmon from Thursday dinner		
Salmon en Papilotte	Vegetarian Vegetable Bolognese	Corn-Crusted Trout with Grilled Vegetables and Potatoes	Chicken Cotoletta with Roasted Carrots and Green Beans
Make double portion of salmon for Friday lunch.	Make double for Saturday lunch. Can make this recipe ahead for a busy night.		

Grocery List Week Four

Notes

Groceries are based on meals for four people. There is enough oatmeal for 3 breakfasts, 2 slices of toast for 3 breakfasts and 1 lunch. Ingredients are not included for side vegetables on Tuesday and Wednesday supper or Thursday and Friday lunch. Make sure to add ingredients to your shopping list for these extra items.

Produce	Quantity
*Fruit for breakfast smoothies and snacks	
*Extra produce for four meals	
Red, Yellow, or Orange Bell Pepper	9
Cherry Tomatoes	1 cup
Cucumber	1
Radish	1 bunch (3 to 4)
Green Beans	11 cups
Avocado	1
Lemon	3
Lime	2
Green Onion	1 bunch
Shallots	2
Garlic	4 cloves
Fennel Bulb	2 medium
Celery	1 bunch (4 stalks)
Carrot	6 large
Kale	4 large leaves
Spinach	8 cups
Small new or red potatoes	4 cups
Fresh Cilantro	1 bunch
Fresh Parsley	1 bunch
Fresh Dill	1 bunch
Fresh Ginger	Small piece

Dairy	Quantity
Old Cheddar Cheese	2 to 3 oz
Lactose-free Yogurt	1 tbsp
Mayonnaise (or Vegenaise)	As needed

Meat & Alternatives	Quantity
Ground Turkey (can use chicken instead)	2 lbs
Ground Beef (lean), Chicken, Turkey or Tempeh (for Vegetable Bolognese)	2 lbs or 4 blocks Tempeh
Chicken, Shrimp, or Tofu (for Peanut Noodle Bowl)	1 lb
Chicken Breast, Boneless, Skinless	500-600 g (at least 2 breasts)
Trout	1.5 lbs
Salmon	3 lbs
Lentils (canned)	2 cans (3 cups)
Egg	3 (plus more for breakfast)
Sunflower or sesame seeds	¼ cup

*Nuts and seeds for snacks

Grains	Quantity
Oatmeal	About 6 cups
Gluten Free Bread	32 slices (≈8 slices/person)
Gluten free buns	8
Soba or Rice Noodles	1 package (250-300 g)
Gluten Free Tortillas, Large	8
Cornmeal	½ cup
Brown or Wild Rice Blend	1 ½ cups
Gluten Free Pasta	½ lbs (dry)
Corn flour	¼ cup
Rice flour	½ cup
Gluten Free Breadcrumbs	1 cup

*Extra wraps or rice paper for Friday lunch

Other	Quantity
White Wine	*optional
Red Wine	*optional
Pureed Tomatoes (Passata)	2 cans
Sliced Almonds	2 tbsp

*Additional items that have not been calculated into the shopping list.
Calculate how many of each you will need for your family depending on your likes, dislikes, meals, and snacks.

Pantry List

There are a few items that you should always have in your pantry as staples so that you can add flavour to your meals without using the common flavours of garlic and onion as these can be major triggers to digestive symptoms. Here is a list of flavour-building ingredients that belong in your pantry or fridge that you will need for the recipes and meal plans.

NOTE: *most oils, vinegars, herbs and spices lose their flavour after about 6 months, so store with care, and replace as needed.*

Oils & Flavourings

- Olive Oil
- Sesame Oil
- White Wine Vinegar
- Balsamic Vinegar
- Apple Cider Vinegar
- Rice Vinegar
- Maple Syrup
- Brown or white sugar
- Tamari (GF)
- Tahini
- Natural Peanut Butter
- Liquid Smoke

Herbs & Spices

- Dried Thyme
- Dried Parsley
- Dried Basil
- Dried Oregano
- Dried Rosemary
- Dried Sage
- Dried Cilantro
- Red Pepper Flakes
- Chili Pepper
- Cayenne
- Smoked Paprika
- Cumin
- Ground Ginger
- Ground Coriander
- Fresh ground salt & pepper

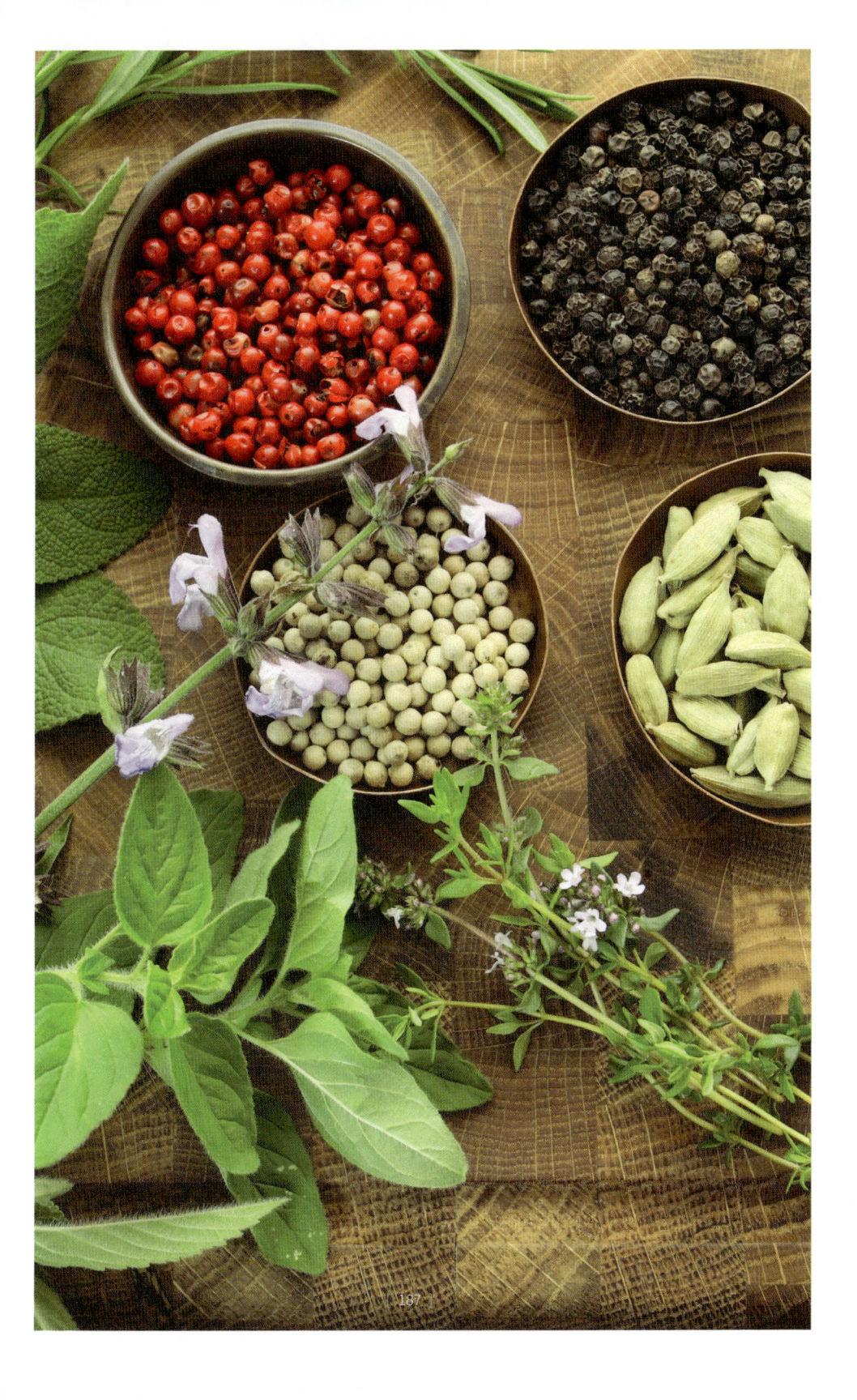

Make Your Own Meal Plan Tool

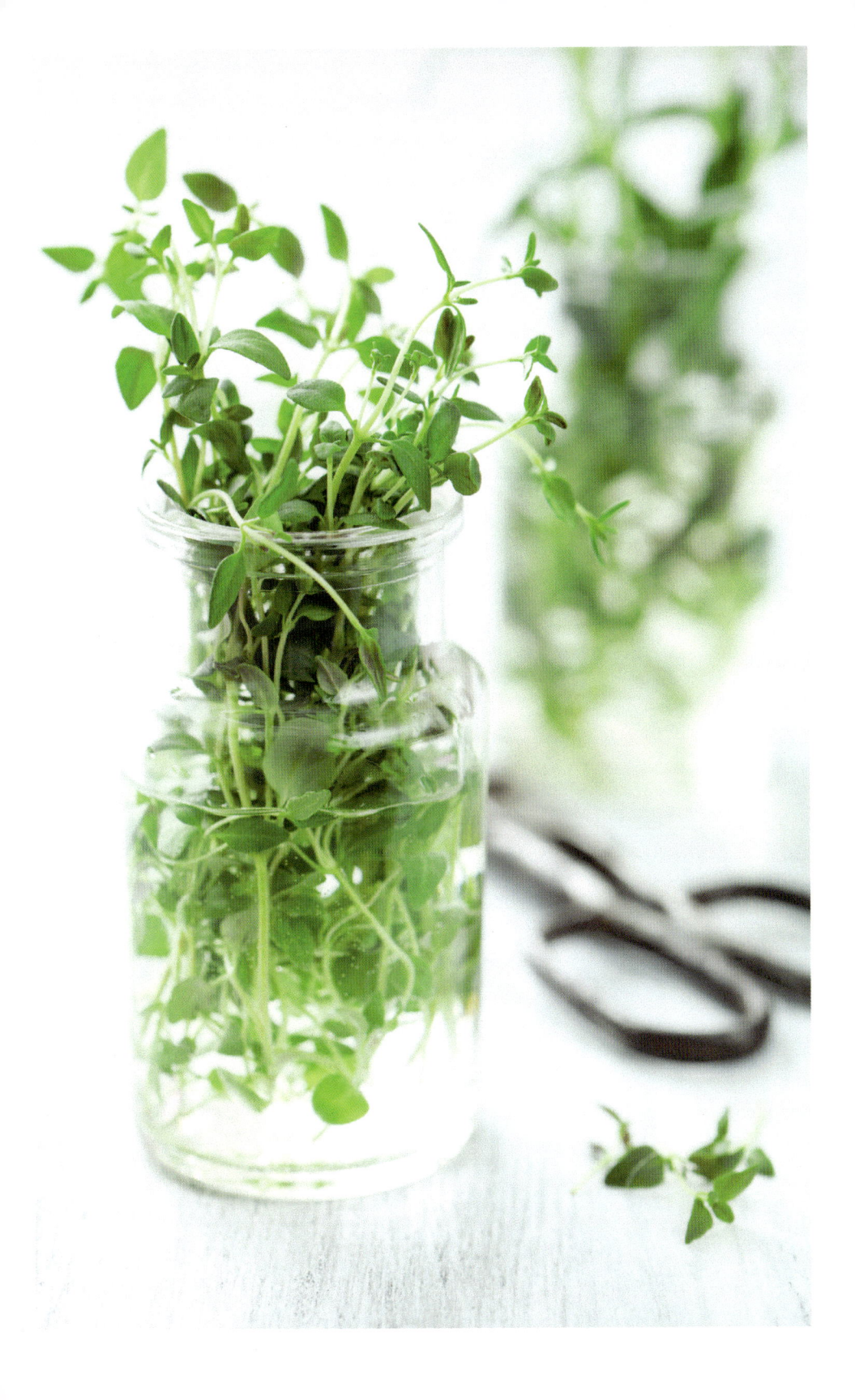

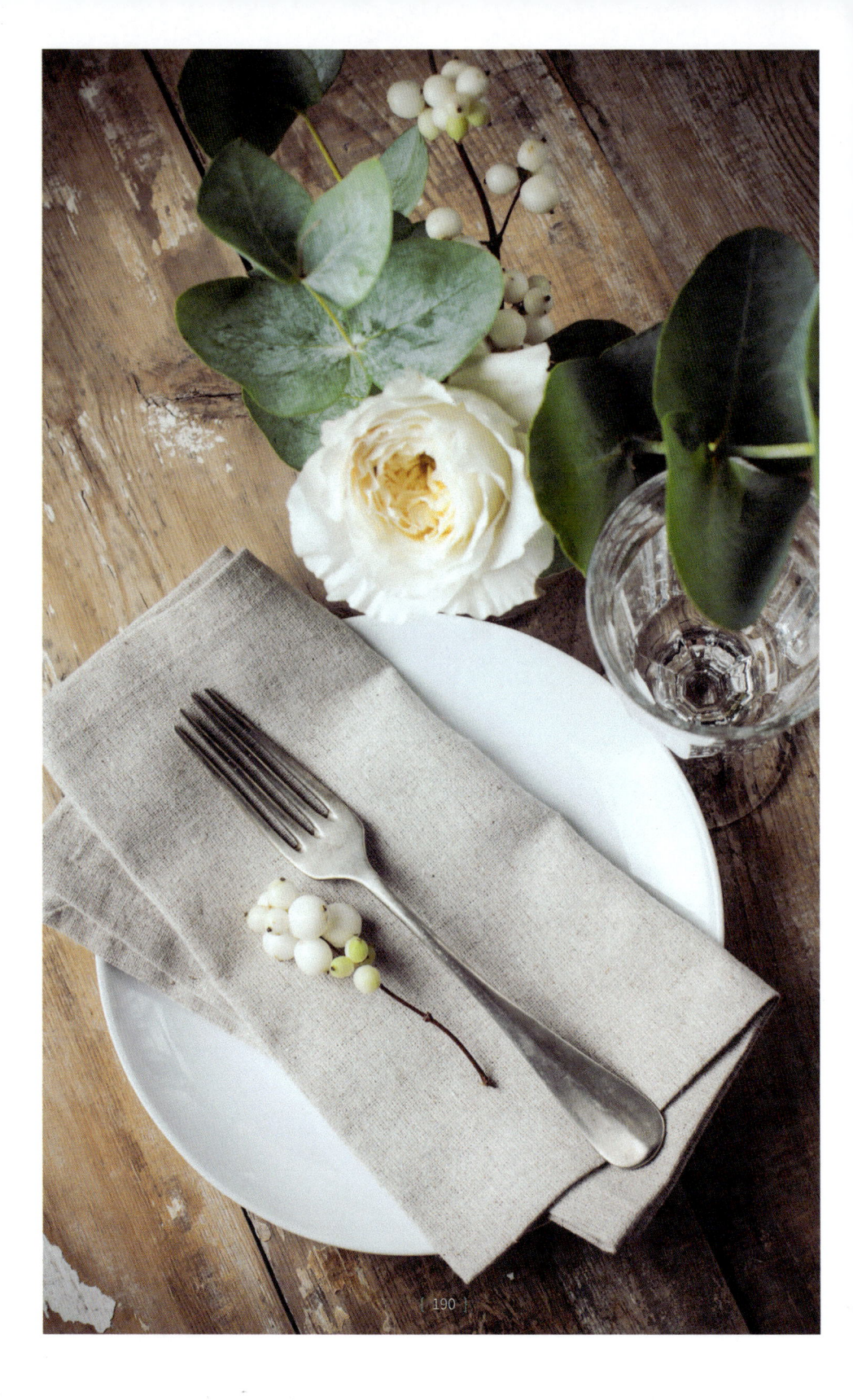

Make-Your-Own Meal Plan

Get ready, Get set, Go!

Do you suffer from IBS or digestive issues like gas, bloating, abdominal pain, diarrhea, or constipation? A digestive diet including low FODMAP foods may help. Let me show you how to eat balanced and fuel your body to balance your blood sugars, provide you with the energy you need, and support your digestive system with foods that are easier to digest.

This Meal Plan template will show you how to organize your meals and snacks in a week. Use this tool along with chapter one and two of this book to create a week of healthy, balanced, gut-friendly foods.

Remember, an exclusion diet like the low FODMAP diet should be followed with the support of a registered dietitian that specializes in digestive nutrition. This Make-Your-Own Meal plan tool is designed to support you in this journey from digestive distress to living your life again!

For more information or if you are looking for coaching and support for digestive distress, please contact us at the Clairmont Digestive Clinic. We would love to help you in your journey to health!

Much love, health, & good eating,
Stephanie Clairmont, MHSc, RD

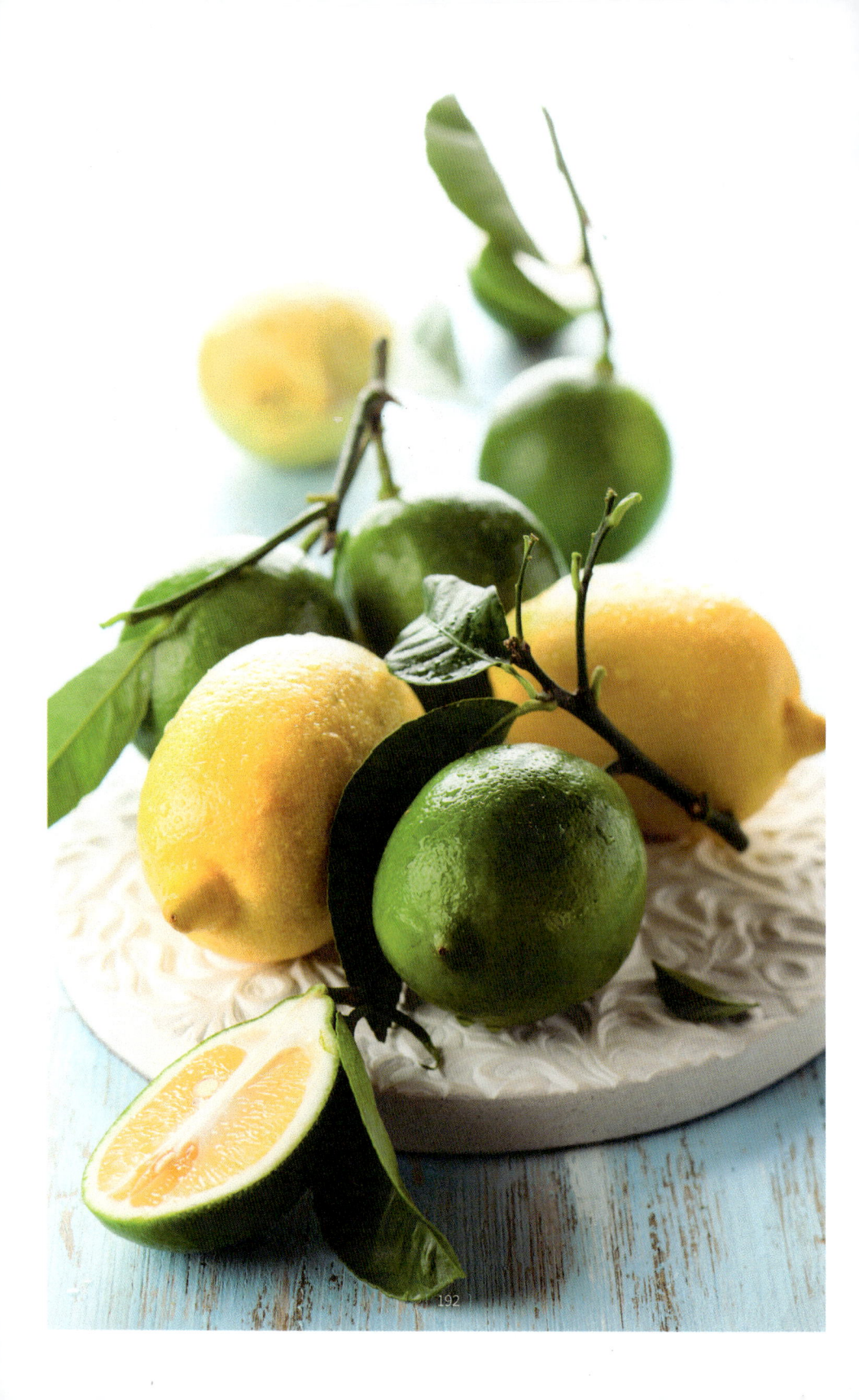

6 Meal Planning Strategies

1. Try to **eat seasonally** the best you can. Choosing seasonal produce, fish, and seafood allows you to eat only the freshest and most nutrient dense foods. Choose local foods as much as possible.

2. Have a variety of breakfasts or choose your favourites to have more often. Make sure you **include a protein every morning** as suggested in the breakfast options. Include at least one cup of almond milk in the morning to provide you with the calcium you need.

3. Choose recipes you can cook ahead for lunch or **double a recipe** from the night before and bring leftovers. Consider choosing lunch recipes that can use leftover chicken—like a quesadilla, rice paper roll, or salad.

4. Consider making double portions at dinner and **freeze leftovers** for lunch or dinner the following week for a healthy meal in a hurry. Most of the meals freeze very well, however avoid freezing gluten-free pasta as it can go quite mushy.

5. For those that have very little time during the week choose quick recipes OR **prepare some foods ahead of time** on the weekend. Wash and prepare fruits and vegetables when you get home from the market and consider making a few items on Sunday and freezing for the week.

6. The plan has been designed for you to enjoy a variety of meat, fish, and meat-free dishes. In one week choose recipes that have different grains/starches and **limit the amount of "gluten-free" foods** like crackers, cookies, noodles, bread, etc. you have to once per day.

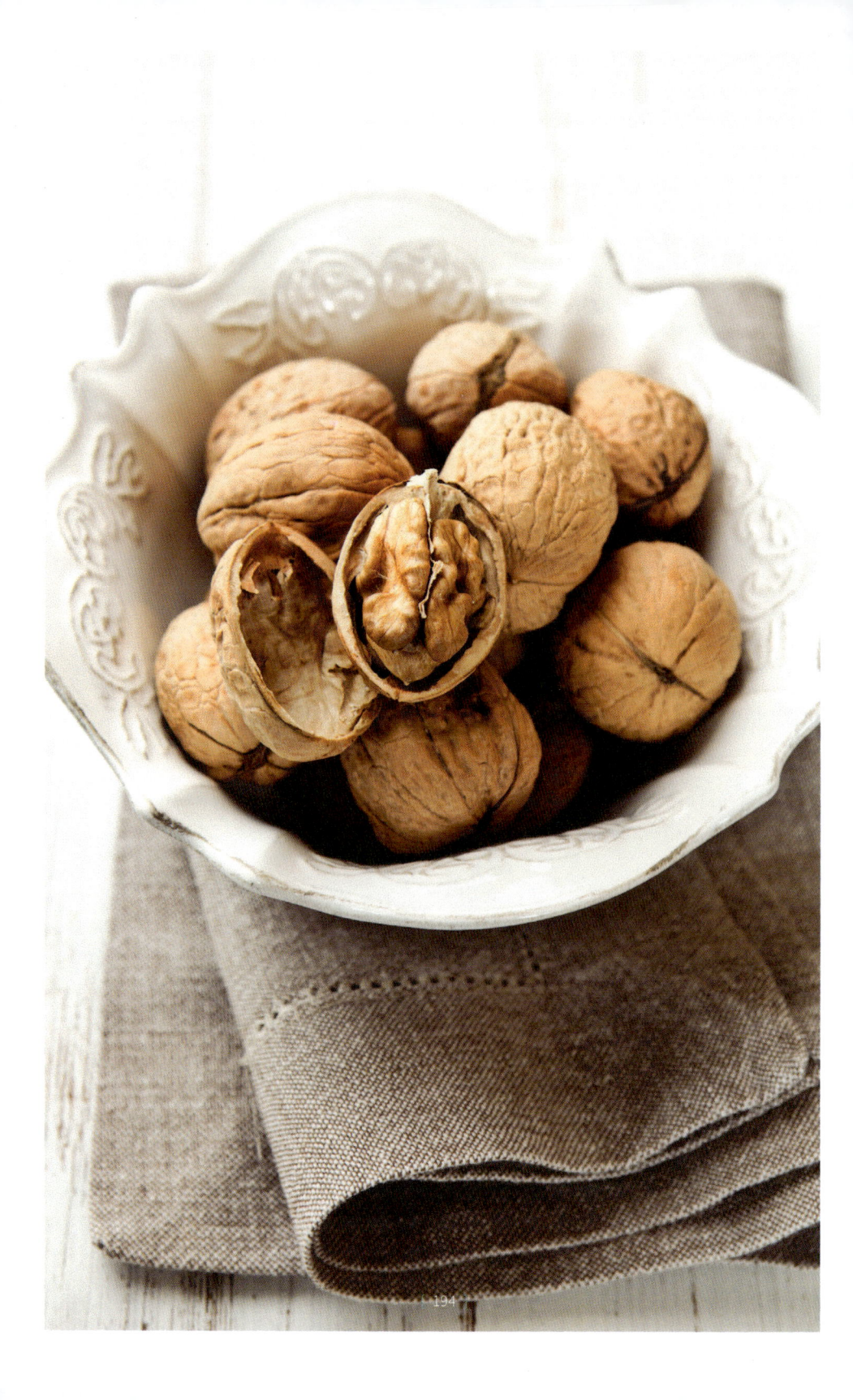

Snack Options

Eat throughout the day. Plan meals and snacks 2 to 4 hours apart to allow your digestive system to work properly – snacking all the time can interfere with your natural digestive process. If you prefer not to snack, avoid periods of time longer than 5 to 6 hours without eating. Eating frequently through the day will help to balance your blood sugar, prevent you from crashing, curb your appetite, and prevent cravings. Choose easily digested, low FODMAP fruit and a protein for a balanced snack.

Choose seasonal produce as often as possible.

SNACKS =

LOW FODMAP FRUIT *(or other low FODMAP carbohydrate)*
+ LOW FODMAP PROTEIN

Snack #1: 1 orange + ¼ cup of walnuts

Snack #2: 1 banana + 2 tbsp peanut butter

Snack #3: 1 cup diced cantaloupe + 3 tbsp hemp seeds sprinkled on top

Snack #4: 1 cup strawberries + ½ cup lactose-free plain yogurt (like Biobest or Liberte brand) *optional pinch of brown sugar

Snack #5: 1 cup blueberries + ½ cup lactose-free cottage cheese

Snack #6: ½ cup grapes + 1 oz (30 g) lactose-free OR old cheese (like cheddar, some Swiss cheese, some Gouda cheese)

Snack #7: 2 Clementine's + ¼ cup sunflower or pumpkin seeds

Make-Your-Own Meal Plan Template

	MONDAY	TUESDAY	WEDNESDAY
Breakfast	Balanced Breakfast *See IBS Master Plan Cookbook section	Balanced Breakfast *See IBS Master Plan Cookbook section	Balanced Breakfast *See IBS Master Plan Cookbook section
Snack	Choose a snack OR create your own	Choose a snack OR create your own	Choose a snack OR create your own
Lunch	Poultry i.e. chicken salad sandwich	Vegetarian i.e. leftover quesadilla	Vegetarian i.e. leafy salad and quinoa
Snack	Choose a snack OR create your own	Choose a snack OR create your own	Choose a snack OR create your own
Supper	Vegetarian i.e. lentil quesadilla	Fish i.e. grilled with salad	Poultry i.e. turkey, potato wedges, & steamed broccoli

The IBS MASTER PLAN

Stephanie CLAIRMONT, RD

THURSDAY	FRIDAY	SATURDAY	SUNDAY
Balanced Breakfast *See IBS Master Plan Cookbook section	Balanced Breakfast *See IBS Master Plan Cookbook section	Balanced Breakfast *See IBS Master Plan Cookbook section	Balanced Breakfast *See IBS Master Plan Cookbook section
Choose a snack OR create your own	Choose a snack OR create your own	Choose a snack OR create your own	Choose a snack OR create your own
Poultry i.e. leftovers from dinner	Vegetarian i.e. Noodle bowl with chickpeas	Vegetarian i.e. roasted vegetable lentil salad	Vegetarian or Fish i.e. tuna pasta salad
Choose a snack OR create your own	Choose a snack OR create your own	Choose a snack OR create your own	Choose a snack OR create your own
Vegetarian i.e. Pasta with tempeh tomato sauce	Fish i.e. breaded with quinoa stir-fry	Meat i.e. GF sausages with rice and grilled peppers	Poultry i.e. turkey burgers with salad

My Meal Plan

Week of:

	MONDAY	TUESDAY	WEDNESDAY
Breakfast			
Snack			
Lunch			
Snack			
Supper			

THURSDAY	FRIDAY	SATURDAY	SUNDAY

About the Author

STEPHANIE CLAIRMONT, MHSC, RD

Culinary Dietitian

Owner, Clairmont Digestive Clinic

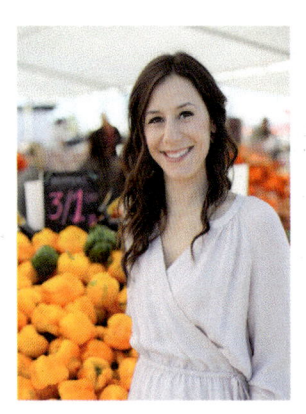

Stephanie Clairmont is a Culinary Dietitian, Digestive Nutrition Expert, and Entrepreneur living and working in Southern Ontario. She completed a Bachelor of Applied Science undergraduate degree from the University of Guelph in 2005 and then completed a Master of Health Science degree in Community Nutrition from the University of Toronto in 2009. Stephanie also completed culinary training at Liaison College in 2011. She is a current member of the College of Dietitians of Ontario and Dietitians of Canada.

After months of discomfort and an unexpected change in digestion, Stephanie was diagnosed with Irritable Bowel Syndrome (IBS) and Hiatus Hernia in 2007. As she did research on the best evidence-based practices to improve symptoms for herself, she realized the growing number of people in her practice as well as around the world suffering from IBS. She found that so many people just didn't realize they could actually feel better with whole health strategies. With a passion for good food and to help others, Stephanie founded the Clairmont Digestive Clinic in 2012.

Stephanie believes that real, wholesome food is the true key to health, from the way food is grown, all the way to how it is presented on the plate. Stephanie has been teaching cooking classes in a variety of settings since 2001 and continues to teach clients and health professional how nutritious food can also be delicious. She incorporates recipes, cooking techniques, and local food discussions into her daily practice. She supports clients in their quest to eat sustainable, seasonal, and delicious food, while being healthy. Stephanie is passionate about showing people living with exclusions due to allergies, intolerances, IBS, and other digestive issues that food can still be absolutely delicious!

Keep in Touch!

Follow Stephanie:

- https://www.facebook.com/glutenfreeitalian
- https://twitter.com/theIBSdietitian
- http://instagram.com/theibsdietitian
- https://www.youtube.com/stephanieclairmont
- http://www.pinterest.com/stephclairmont/
- **Blog:** http://stephanieclairmont.com/blog/